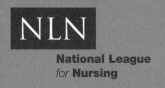

National League
for **Nursing**

INTERPROFESSIONAL EDUCATION AND COLLABORATIVE PRACTICE

CREATING A BLUEPRINT FOR NURSE EDUCATORS

Edited by:

Elizabeth Speakman, EdD, RN, CDE, FNAP, ANEF

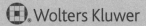

. Wolters Kluwer

Philadelphia • Baltimore • New York • London
Buenos Aires • Hong Kong • Sydney • Tokyo

Executive Editor: Sherry Dickinson
Product Director: Jennifer K. Forestieri
Development Editor: Meredith L. Brittain
Production Project Manager: Marian Bellus
Design Coordinator: Terry Mallon
Illustration Coordinator: Jennifer Clements
Manufacturing Coordinator: Karin Duffield
Marketing Manager: Todd McQueston
Prepress Vendor: Aptara, Inc.

Library of Congress Cataloging-in-Publication Data

Names: Speakman, Elizabeth, editor. | National League for Nursing, issuing
 body.
Title: Interprofessional education and collaborative practice : creating a
 blueprint for nurse educators / edited by Elizabeth Speakman.
Description: Philadelphia : National League for Nursing ; Wolters Kluwer,
 [2017] | Includes bibliographical references.
Identifiers: LCCN 2016027242 | ISBN 9781934758236
Subjects: | MESH: Education, Nursing | Interprofessional Relations |
 Cooperative Behavior | Teaching–methods
Classification: LCC RT71 | NLM WY 18 | DDC 610.73071/1–dc23
LC record available at https://lccn.loc.gov/2016027242

DRC0816

www.LWW.com   www.NLN.org

About the Editor

Elizabeth Speakman, EdD, RN, CDE, FNAP, ANEF is the Codirector of the Jefferson Center for Interprofessional Education [JCIPE] and a Professor of Nursing at Thomas Jefferson University. Dr. Speakman has been an educator for thirty-one years and prior to her current post, Dr. Speakman was associate dean of student affairs and assistant dean of the RN-BSN program in the Jefferson College of Nursing. Dr. Speakman is a fellow in the Academy of Nursing Education, a fellow in the National Academies of Practice and a Robert Wood Johnson Foundation Executive Nurse Fellow Alumnus and is nationally known for her work on faculty and curriculum development and interprofessional education with over 100 national and international presentations.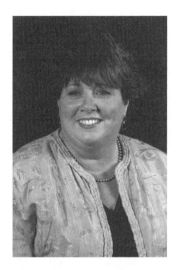

Dr. Speakman is the recipient of the Dean's Faculty Achievement Award for excellence in teaching, research and service and the prestigious Louise McManus Medal for distinguished service from Teachers College, Columbia University. Dr. Speakman has served as Johnson and Johnson and a Jonas Foundation Faculty Mentor and in 2014 was inducted into the Hall of Fame, at Teachers College, Columbia University. Dr. Speakman served two consecutive 3-year terms as a Board of Governor for the National League for Nursing and serves as both an editorial board member as well as a peer review member for several publications that focus on nursing education, interprofessional education and collaborative practice. Dr. Speakman serves as a consultant to many national organizations aiding them in implementing interprofessional education and collaborative practice initiatives.

Dr. Speakman received her bachelor's degree in nursing from New York's Wagner College in 1980; her master's and doctoral degrees in education from Columbia University in 1985 and 2000, respectively; and a certificate in healthcare education from the Harvard-Macy Institute at Harvard University.

About the Contributors

Christine Arenson, MD is the codirector of the Jefferson Center for Interprofessional Education at Thomas Jefferson University. Dr. Arenson graduated from the University of Delaware in 1986 and Jefferson Medical College in 1990. She completed family medicine residency training at Thomas Jefferson University Hospital, serving as chief resident in 1993, followed by a fellowship in geriatric medicine. She is a professor and interim chair of the Department of Family and Community Medicine. Her interests are in geriatric medicine, interprofessional education, and collaborative practice models.

Anne R. Bavier, PhD, RN, FAAN is a nationally recognized healthcare leader who has held posts at top-ranked universities and at the National Institutes of Health. Prior to becoming dean of the University of Texas at Arlington (UTA) College of Nursing in August 2014, she was dean of the University of Connecticut School of Nursing and dean of nursing at Saint Xavier University in Chicago.

Under her leadership, UTA's College of Nursing and Health Innovation has been named a National League for Nursing Center of Excellence in Nursing Education, one of only 12 nursing schools in the nation to earn the designation this year. Dr. Bavier earned an undergraduate nursing degree from Duke University, a Master of Nursing degree from Emory University, and a doctoral degree from Duquesne University.

In addition to her experience in higher education, she worked as a program director in the National Institutes of Health's National Cancer Institute and as deputy director of the agency's Office of Research on Women's Health. She is president of the National League for Nursing and has authored or coauthored numerous publications on nursing education, professional development, and oncology nursing.

Dr. Bavier is a fellow of the American Academy of Nursing and the Institute of Medicine of Chicago and was the first recipient of the Edith Moore Copeland Founder's Award for Creativity from the Sigma Theta Tau International Honor Society of Nursing. She also received the NIH Director's Award from the National Institutes of Health and the Administrator's Award while at the Agency for Health Care Policy and Research. Both awards are the highest honors given by these agencies. Dr. Bavier is also the recipient of the Legion of Honor Gold Medallion from the Philadelphia-based Chapel of Four Chaplains.

Mary T. Bouchaud, PhD, MSN, CNS, RN, CRRN is an assistant professor and the community clinical coordinator for the Jefferson College of Nursing. Dr. Bouchaud graduated from Capella University with her doctorate in community, social work, and geriatrics. For the past 7 years, Dr. Bouchaud has been working closely with the Jefferson College of Interprofessional Education (JCIPE) department, integrating interprofessional collaborative education strategies to prepare prelicensure second-degree and traditional baccalaureate nursing students for nursing practice in the 21st century. Teaching strategies include narrative pedagogy and unfolding case scenarios analyzed by interprofessional student groups followed by an interprofessional panel for post case reflection to stimulate classroom discourse and the formation and inclusion of interprofessional clinical teams in community clinical sites, such as state and federal prisons, home care visits, and wellness centers. Dr. Bouchaud has coauthored several articles and copresented with JCIPE on interprofessional education and collaborative practice models at professional conferences.

Lauren Collins, MD is an associate professor of Family and Community Medicine and Geriatrics at Thomas Jefferson University, associate director of Jefferson's Center for Interprofessional Education (JCIPE), and director of Jefferson's Health Mentors Program. In 2015, she was selected as one of five recipients of the Macy Faculty Scholars Program from the Josiah Macy Jr. Foundation. In addition, she has received the American Academy of Family Physicians' Award for Excellence in Graduate Medical Education, Jefferson's IPE Education Award, three AAMC/Macy Collaborative Development Awards, and a Health Resources and Services Administration (HRSA) Geriatric Academic Career Award. Dr. Collins has served as principal investigator of a 5-year HRSA-funded undergraduate medical education grant, *The Jefferson Patient-Centered Medical Home (PCMH) Predoctoral Education Project*. Dr. Collins serves as a peer reviewer and/or editorial board member for six peer-reviewed journals, has more than 20 peer-reviewed publications and more than 50 national presentations, teaches and advises students, and serves on multiple committees for interprofessional education (IPE). Dr. Collins' career focus and passion is for IPE, curricular innovation, and scholarship. Dr. Collins received her undergraduate degree with honors from Princeton University, and she completed her medical degree at Jefferson Medical College and a family medicine residency and geriatric medicine fellowship at Thomas Jefferson University Hospital in Philadelphia.

Sarah Dallas, BA is the education coordinator for the Jefferson Center for Interprofessional Education at Thomas Jefferson University. In this role, Ms. Dallas oversees the day-to-day operations of the Health Mentors Program. This involves volunteer recruitment, interfacing with Jefferson students, and organizing large group meetings. Ms. Dallas graduated from Fordham University with a major in sociology.

John J. Duffy, DNP, MSN, RN, CCRN is an assistant professor in the College of Public Health-Nursing at Temple University. Formerly the director of Nursing Simulation and Clinical Skills at Thomas Jefferson University, Dr. Duffy is a graduate of Temple University, where he earned his Bachelor of Science in nursing. He later earned his master's degree from Widener University as a clinical nurse specialist in burns/emergency and trauma and completed his doctor of nursing practice degree at Case Western Reserve University. He served as a burn nurse in the U.S. Navy in Saudi Arabia during Desert Storm #1, and his research interests are high-fidelity simulation as a teaching pedagogy, validated checklist for clinical skills, interprofessional education, teamwork and communication, and patient safety.

Tracey Vause Earland, PhD (c), MS, OTR/L is an assistant professor in the Department of Occupational Therapy at Thomas Jefferson University in Philadelphia. For more than 20 years, she has served as a research interventionist and project coordinator on various funded studies centered on the frail elderly, dementia management and family caregiving, low vision rehab, and community reintegration for veterans with mild head injury. Ms. Earland is a faculty member of Jefferson's Center for Interprofessional Education and currently serves as the codirector of the Jefferson Health Mentors Program.

Alan T. Forstater, MD, FACEP is an assistant professor in the Department of Emergency Medicine at Thomas Jefferson University. He has been an emergency medicine attending physician and educator for 37 years and is board certified in emergency medicine and internal medicine. He loves teaching students of all ages and levels of training. He has a special interest in communication skills, professionalism, patient safety, and team training. He teaches these skills locally and at national meetings and is a master trainer in TeamSTEPPS®. He has been recognized for his patient care and contributions to education, specifically his contribution to interprofessional education at Jefferson.

Carolyn Giordano, PhD is the director of the Office of Institutional Research at Thomas Jefferson University, an assistant professor of biostatistics for the Jefferson College of Pharmacy, and a researcher with the Jefferson Center for Interprofessional Education. She has a doctoral degree in educational and experimental psychology and more than 15 years of experience conducting research in health science and medical education. She has numerous publications on interprofessional education and has spoken widely on that topic as well.

Mary Hanson-Zalot, EdD, MSN, RN, AOCN, CNE is the director of the FACT and RN-BSN programs at Thomas Jefferson University's Jefferson College of Nursing. She graduated from Holy Family University with a bachelor's degree in nursing and earned a master's degree from Gwynedd-Mercy College with a clinical specialty in oncology and a functional role in nursing education. She is a doctoral candidate at Widener University in higher education and administrative leadership. Research interests of Ms. Hanson-Zalot include enhancement of the adjunct faculty role in nursing education, second-degree student learning in nursing education, and innovative teaching strategies. She was named as the 2013-2014 recipient of the James B. Erdmann, PhD, Award for Excellence in Interprofessional Education and was a 2009 fellow for leadership in academic nursing programs of the AACN. She serves on the Board of Delta Rho, Jefferson's Chapter of STTI. She is a member of Omicron Delta Kappa, Kappa Delta Pi, the Association of American Colleges and Universities, the American Association of Critical-Care Nurses, the Oncology Nursing Society, and the National League for Nursing.

Shelley Cohen Konrad, PhD, LCSW, FNAP is a professor and interim director of the University of New England (UNE) School of Social Work and director of UNE's Interprofessional Education Collaborative. Dr. Cohen Konrad has 30 years of clinical social work experience serving children, families, and communities. She developed two nonprofits that provide low-barrier child and family resources to individuals and families across Maine. Her book *Child and Family Practice: A Relational Perspective* was published in 2013 by Lyceum. Over the past 10 years, Dr. Cohen Konrad has established a national reputation as an educator and advocate for interprofessional and collaborative practice education. She has published widely on these topics in peer-reviewed journals and serves as an associate editor for the *Journal of Interprofessional Care*.

Kevin J. Lyons, PhD, FASAHP is a research consultant in the Office of Institutional Research at Thomas Jefferson University. Dr. Lyons has presented numerous papers at national and international scientific meetings and has been a frequent consultant to universities and government agencies on issues such as research development and program improvement. He has published numerous articles in peer-reviewed journals and has made more than 170 scholarly presentations to local, national, and international audiences. He coauthored the book *Successful: Grant Writing: Strategies for Health and Human Services Professionals*, the fourth edition of which was recently published by Springer. Dr. Lyons has written chapters for the books *Medicine and Health Care into the 21st Century, Leadership in Rural Health: Interprofessional Education and Practice*, and *Allied Education, Practice Issues and Trends into the 21st Millennium*. For 10 years, Dr. Lyons served as an editor of the *Journal of Allied Health* and has received the J. Warren Perry Distinguished Author Award and been elected as a fellow in that organization. He coedited a special issue of the journal, published in September 2010 on interprofessional education, which featured papers from national and international leaders in the field. Dr Lyons is one of the founding members of the International Association for Interprofessional Education and Collaborative Practice and the American Interprofessional Health Collaborative.

Chelsea Gorman Lytle, BSN, RN is a perioperative nurse at Vanderbilt University Medical Center. She first encountered the concepts of interprofessional education (IPE) and collaborative practice while attending Thomas Jefferson University's Jefferson School of Nursing. During her time at Jefferson, she worked with other health professions students to establish Jefferson Students for Interprofessional Education (JSIPE) and developed and implemented an extracurricular interprofessional initiative to improve the clinical relevance of IPE. After completing her bachelor's degree in nursing in 2015, Ms. Lytle moved to Nashville, where she works as a perioperative nurse at Vanderbilt University Medical Center.

Trisha A. Mason, MA is the service-learning coordinator and an adjunct professor in Westbrook College of Health Professions at the University of New England. Ms. Mason received her bachelor's degree in world politics from Hamilton College and her master's degree in public policy and administration from the Muskie School at the University of Southern Maine. Prior to moving back to her home state of Maine, Trisha spent 5 years in Washington, DC, at the Institute of International Education, supporting a global business student adviser program, and at the U.S. Chamber of Commerce, where she led U.S. congressional delegation visits to Latin America, orchestrated head of state visits, and managed an ambassador tour in collaboration with the Brazilian Embassy. While in graduate school, she worked at the Maine Small Business Development Centers overseeing a federal demonstration project. Fluent in Spanish and having traveled extensively to more than 30 countries for both personal and professional pursuits, Ms. Mason first joined the University of New England in 2006 to establish its study abroad program. In 2011, still at University of New England, Trisha went on to build a service-learning program for health professions students by creating mutually beneficial local partnerships and supporting logistics for the university's Cross Cultural Health Immersion Program in Ghana. While trying to keep up with her 3-year-old twin girls, Ms. Mason also enjoys cooking global cuisine that she has discovered through her travels and taking in all of the wonderful outdoor adventures the great state of Maine has to offer.

Catherine Mills joined the Jefferson Center for Interprofessional Education (JCIPE) team in 1997 as their administrative assistant. At the JCIPE, she supports the codirectors of the program, the assistant director, the education coordinator, and the program assistant. Besides her other duties, she coordinates the biannual conference for the center, which has nearly 150 participants. Prior to joining the JCIPE, Ms. Mills began her career in the Department of Family and Community Medicine at Thomas Jefferson University in 1990. She supported three family medicine physicians. In 1995, she became the fellowship coordinator for the directors of the faculty development, geriatric medicine, and sports medicine fellowships in addition to her administrative assistant duties for the department.

Jennifer Morton, DNP, MPH is an associate professor in and the chair of the Department of Nursing at the University of New England. Dr. Morton's scholarship resides in public health nursing and advancing outcomes for vulnerable communities. She leads health-related immersion experiences in Ghana for interprofessional teams of students and faculty while having cultivated relationships with the Ghana Health Service and local universities. Most recently, she was the principal investigator on a Health Resources and Services Administration Nurse Education, Practice, Quality and Retention grant focused on improving the health of immigrant and refugee communities through innovations in team-based care.

Dimitrios Papanagnou, MD, MPH, EdD (c) is an emergency medicine physician and vice chair for education in the Department of Emergency Medicine at Thomas Jefferson University Hospital in Philadelphia. He is also the assistant dean for faculty development at the Sidney Kimmel Medical College of Thomas Jefferson University. Dr. Papanagnou graduated from the New York University (NYU) School of Medicine. As a Josiah Macy Jr. Foundation Scholar, he received a master's degree in public health at Columbia University and then completed his residency in emergency medicine at the NYU/Bellevue Hospital Center. Dr. Papanagnou is now in the final stages of completing a doctoral degree in adult education at Columbia University.

Karen T. Pardue, PhD, RN, CNE, ANEF is the associate dean for academic affairs in the Westbrook College of Health Professions at the University of New England (UNE). Her expertise focuses on nursing education and interprofessional education (IPE) curriculum development and evaluation. Dr. Pardue provided leadership in the design and implementation of UNE's innovative undergraduate IPE coursework. For a decade, she provided leadership to a novel international academic partnership involving UNE and the Israel College in Tel Aviv. She is active with the National League for Nursing (NLN), chairing the Task Group on Innovation in Nursing Education, the Academy of Nursing Education Selection Committee, and serving as a mentor for the Johnson and Johnson/NLN Faculty Mentoring Program. Nominated in 2013 by the governor of Maine, she serves on the New England Board of Higher Education, where she currently chairs the Maine delegation. Dr. Pardue was inducted as a fellow in the Academy of Nursing

Education in 2007. She has grant-funded projects from the Health Resources and Services Administration, the Arthur Vining Davis Foundations, and the Josiah Macy Jr. Foundation, addressing IPE models and collaborative nursing leadership.

Anne Marie Pettit, MSN, RN graduated from Abington Memorial Hospital School of Nursing in 1983, LaSalle University with her BSN in 1993, and Villanova University with her Masters in Nursing Education in 2005. She has been a Critical Care Nurse for 33 years and a Nurse Educator for 12 years, specializing in the use of Simulation in Nursing education. She has presented locally and nationally on the use of simulation with student nurses. She currently works as a Nursing Professional Development Specialist at Good Shepherd Penn Partners, The Specialty Hospital at Rittenhouse in Philadelphia.

Kathryn M. Shaffer, EdD, MSN, RN, CNE has been a full-time faculty member since 2007 and currently is the director of clinical education and faculty development at Thomas Jefferson University's Jefferson College of Nursing. Ms. Shaffer is a graduate of the Jefferson School of Nursing and received her Master of Science in nursing with a concentration in nursing education from Mansfield University. She received her doctorate in education from the University of Delaware, where she focused her studies on technology and higher education. Ms. Shaffer's interest in education and technology has led to several innovative teaching strategies, which she has presented both regionally and nationally on cultivating the next generation of nurses. She is an active faculty member in Jefferson's Center for Interprofessional Education and has transformed clinical teaching rounds. She recently became involved in the Telehealth Initiative at Thomas Jefferson University Hospital to create a National Academic Center for Telehealth Medicine.

Shoshana Sicks, EdM, AB, EdD (s) is the assistant director of the Jefferson Center for Interprofessional Education at Thomas Jefferson University. She has extensive experience in higher education administration, including student and curricular affairs, program and curriculum development and management, international education and global health, and interprofessional education. Shoshana received a bachelor's degree in Spanish from Bowdoin College and a master's degree in higher education administration from Harvard University.

Elena M. Umland, PharmD, BS is an associate dean for academic affairs and a professor of pharmacy practice in the Jefferson College of Pharmacy (JCP) at Thomas Jefferson University in Philadelphia. She has held elected leadership positions for the American Association of Colleges of Pharmacy (AACP) Women's Faculty SIG (secretary, 2013-2015; president elect, 2015-present), and she is a 2007 graduate of the AACP Academic Leadership Fellows Program. She has served on the AACP Academic Affairs Committee (2014-2015), the communications subcommittee of the Assessment SIG (2011-2013), and the AACP Dean's Task Force on Achieving Institutional Excellence (2009), and she chaired the Sub-Task Force that developed the AACP preceptor survey as a member of the Institutional Research Advisory Committee (2006). Currently, Dr. Umland's primary responsibilities include oversight of JCP's curriculum and the school's assessment plan. Her scholarly activity has focused on women's health issues and has expanded to include presentation of assessment activities, with an increasing focus on interprofessional education, at national and international meetings.

Julia M. Ward, PhD, RN is an associate professor at Thomas Jefferson University's Jefferson College of Nursing and has been a nurse educator for 26 years. She is the recipient of the James B. Erdmann Award for Excellence in Interprofessional Education and participates in the interprofessional community at Thomas Jefferson University. Dr. Ward is a member of Jefferson College of Interprofessional Education's Health Mentors Program Faculty Committee and was a cocontributor to the development and implementation of the Jefferson Scale of Attitudes Toward Interprofessional Collaboration (JeffSATIC).

Mayumi A. Willgerodt, PhD, MPH, RN is a professor in the School of Nursing and Health Studies and director of graduate students for the University of Washington (UW) Bothell. Dr. Willgerodt's work is focused in interprofessional education (IPE) and collaborative practice; she has been involved in numerous initiatives within and beyond UW. She has participated and/or led the development of community-based cases for use in IPE, the creation of a longitudinal IPE curricula, and faculty development. She is a member of several grant teams focused on IPE and patient safety and coleads the evaluation core of a Health Resources and Services Administration-funded grant focused on integrating IPE and technology in doctor of nursing practice curriculum at UW. Dr. Willgerodt is a former Macy Faculty Scholar, is on the editorial board of *Journal of School Nursing*, and is associate editor for the *Journal of Interprofessional Education and Practice*.

Brenda K. Zierler, PhD, RN, FAAN is a professor at Biobehavioral Nursing and Health Systems, School of Nursing, University of Washington (UW) and an interprofessional education (IPE) scholar for the UW Health Sciences Center (Inaugural). Dr. Zierler's research explores the relationships between the delivery of healthcare and outcomes at both the patient and system level. Her primary appointment is in the School of Nursing at UW, but she holds three adjunct appointments: two in the School of Medicine and one in the School of Public Health. Currently, Dr. Zierler is co-principal investigator on a Josiah Macy-funded grant with Dr. Les Hall to develop a national train-the-trainer (T3) faculty development program for IPE and collaborative practice (CP). She also leads three Health Resources and Services Administration training grants: one focused on technology-enhanced IPE for advanced practice students, the second focused on interprofessional CP for advanced heart failure patients, and the third training grant focused on an education-practice partnership to improve advanced heart failure training and outcomes for rural and underserved populations in an accountable care organization. Dr. Zierler is the codirector for the UW Center for Health Sciences Interprofessional Education, Practice and Research and director of faculty development for the UW Institute for Simulation and Interprofessional Studies in the School of Medicine. Dr. Zierler is a board member and past chair of the American Interprofessional Health Collaborative, and a member of the Institute of Medicine's Global Forum on Innovation in Health Professions Education.

Foreword

Although there is growing support for interprofessional education (IPE), implementation of collaborative training programs across the continuum of health professions education has generally been slower and more uneven than many advocates would like. Common explanations include the lack of purposeful integration of education with healthcare systems; the absence of well-tested conceptual models linking IPE to learning, health, and system outcomes; and the relative lack of guidance on the design, execution, and evaluation of IPE programs. Indeed, students and their teachers may be poorly prepared for collaborative learning. And the learning environment, especially the clinical workplace, may be less than conducive to collaboration across professions.

As suggested by its title, this book provides a blueprint for adopting IPE and addressing the major opportunities and barriers to the implementation of collaborative practice. The central focus is nursing programs, but medical and allied health disciplines will find much to value as well. Indeed, the messages conveyed have broad utility for all health professions and broad applicability to the wide spectrum of institutions struggling with the implementation of interprofessional learning programs.

The development, execution, and evaluation of interprofessional curricular efforts are covered, with emphasis on the practical considerations that so often bedevil efforts at innovation. Exemplars of success are presented throughout, providing not only models to emulate but also thought experiments for divergent design efforts by others in the future. Interprofessional competency frameworks, conceptual models for evaluating outcomes, evaluation principles, and different venues for interprofessional activities—including classroom, simulation, and experiential opportunities (in traditional, community-based and service-learning sites)—are included. The seminal importance of institutional mobilization, project champions, and faculty development are repeatedly emphasized.

The failure to appropriately value IPE as a key learning modality for the health professions may ultimately stem from a skewed vision of health as being dominated by episodic diagnosis and treatment rather than a lifelong effort aimed at disease prevention and sustaining wellness. Ultimately, achieving "health" is an interactive process among providers, individual persons, families, and communities. As such, it is impossible to get away from the central tenet of IPE—the development of collaborative learning and team care models that support the well-being of individuals and communities alike. Advancing collaboration and teamwork by providing practical wisdom is the goal of this book—a goal that the authors readily achieve. More books like this one will be equally welcome.

Malcolm Cox, MD
Adjunct Professor of Medicine,
Perelman School of Medicine,
University of Pennsylvania
Former Chief Academic Affiliations Officer,
U.S. Department of Veterans Affairs

Preface

The value of high-functioning teams for enhancing patient safety and quality care has led to a renewed interest in the interprofessional education (IPE) and collaborative practice (CP) movement across many health education disciplines. To prepare future healthcare practitioners to practice in this environment, educators need to find meaningful learning opportunities that give students the best experience practicing in teams. However, the incongruent curriculum and accreditation standards, combined with the logistics of class schedules and rotations, have long been and continue to be noted as the greatest impediments to collaborative IPE learning opportunities.

This book is a blueprint designed to assist nurse educators in developing meaningful and purposeful team-based learning opportunities for students. Each chapter, coauthored by a team of interprofessionals, presents a broad perspective of how to create, deliver, and evaluate IPE and CP learning opportunities. The benefit of IPE is that students from a variety of backgrounds and disciplines have the opportunity to practice and effectively communicate with each other. It behooves nurse educators to recognize that nurses will not be able to engage in team-based patient-centered care if they are not given opportunities to practice these skills in the learning environment as a student.

Chapter 1 describes the state of interprofessional learning and creates the context for the nurse educator. By illustrating the history of nursing, the authors help the reader to understand that nurses have always been central to the delivery of patient-centered care. In addition, the chapter highlights specific exemplars of IPE and CP that can be incorporated into nursing curricula.

In Chapter 2, the theoretical and conceptual models that govern IPE are described and placed within the context of IPE and CP. The Interprofessional Education Collaborative (IPEC) Core Competencies threaded throughout the book are discussed in detail in this chapter, giving the reader the ability to construct the "how to initiate" process of developing IPE and CP curricula.

The importance and value in creating a systematic plan to develop faculty IPE and CP expertise is illustrated in Chapter 3. This chapter offers examples that the reader can use to design a faculty development program, and it highlights a specific exemplar from the University of Washington's faculty mentoring program.

With a student (now a graduate) as a coauthor, Chapter 4 focuses on student learning. Adult higher education literature is replete with the notion that to truly understand the impact of the learning experience, learners should describe the experience through their own eyes. This chapter describes the 8-year longitudinal Jefferson Health Mentors Program at Thomas Jefferson University, which matches each team of interprofessional students to a person living in the community with at least one chronic illness. Through a series of activities, students learn how to work to provide team-based approaches to care.

Chapter 5 concentrates on the classroom setting or "IPE didactic content." It describes the impact of culture change that occurs with integrating IPE. Through the IVAN© story (Dr. Mary Bouchaud's father), the reader learns how real life can create wonderful intricate IPE and CP case studies that can be used to prepare students for the experiential clinical arena. This chapter discusses how, within the confines of classroom walls, students who are given an opportunity to dialogue with interprofessional healthcare professionals learn how those multiple professions would care for IVAN using the team-based approach.

In Chapter 6, the authors describe how experiential IPE and CP learning opportunities help students master the four IPEC Core Competencies. This chapter offers numerous clinical exemplars that the reader can use to develop a systematic plan to link IPE with collaborative practice (CP).

Chapter 7 explores the merit of implementing community-based IPE opportunities that promote CP while serving vulnerable underserved populations living in the community. The authors describe a community and a nonacademic health center collaboration exemplar, which provides students with a real-world scenario that develops their teamwork and communication skills and fosters a respect for cultural humility, health literacy, relational connection, and resourcefulness.

Technology and IPE is the focus of Chapter 8. In this chapter, the authors demonstrate how technology can personalize and accelerate learning, as well as support collaboration across health professions. Interspersed throughout the chapter are examples of technological modalities that have the potential to redefine IPE and CP by transforming and creating new paradigms of team-based care.

It has been well established that simulation activities allow learners to repeatedly practice requisite skills and critical decision making without risking harm to patients. In Chapter 9, the authors describe how interprofessional simulation has the added benefit of providing teams of health profession students with opportunities to problem solve through team communication and behavior. Various simulation examples are noted throughout the chapter, and the use of the TeamSTEPPS® as a specific simulation technique is discussed as an exemplar.

Chapter 10 provides a conceptual framework for interprofessional and CP opportunities within the international context. The author describes international interprofessional learning, preparing students to function in multicultural environments while gaining an awareness of other health systems and perspectives in care organization and delivery.

Chapter 11, the final chapter, describes the value and need to create a robust evaluation plan when developing IPE and CP initiatives. In addition, the authors outline the need to disseminate these findings to create a repository of IPE learning activities, as well as to add to the existing IPE and CP body of knowledge and existing literature.

It is evident that the nurse's role on the healthcare team is vital. To that end, it is imperative that nursing students be given the opportunity to engage in IPE and CP learning opportunities. Patients and their families, along with their healthcare providers, will need to work collaboratively to employ strategies that allow patients to "age in place" and be able to self-manage their own chronic and episodic care. Health care in the 21st century will need to have an even greater emphasis on prevention and outpatient/community-based approaches versus the typical inpatient admissions/readmissions cycle. For the healthcare provider of the future, particularly the nurse, the changes in the healthcare delivery system will mean that their respective curricula will need to prepare them to work with other practitioners utilizing team-based models of care.

Elizabeth Speakman, EdD, RN, CDE, FNAP, ANEF
Codirector, Jefferson Center for Interprofessional Education
Professor of Nursing
Thomas Jefferson University
Philadelphia, PA

Acknowledgments

I want to extend my sincere appreciation to the many authors who generously shared their expertise in interprofessional education. Thank you for working collaboratively and truly modeling effective teamwork.

I especially want to acknowledge and thank Mark Laessig and Shoshana Sicks for their attention to detail when reviewing each of the chapters. Thank you to the Robert Wood Johnson Foundation Executive Nurse Fellow Program faculty and staff, as well as my "peeps" Cohort 2012 for encouraging me to take on this project.

A special thank you to Elaine Tagliareni from the National League for Nursing, as well as Sherry Dickerson and Meredith Brittain from Wolters Kluwer, for continuously supporting this endeavor.

Finally, I would like to thank my husband Robert Speakman and children Caroline Speakman and Alexandra Speakman Romano & John Romano—you never doubt and always inspire me to reach.

Elizabeth Speakman, EdD, RN, CDE, FNAP, ANEF

Contents

1

Introduction to Interprofessional Education and Collaborative Practice: Setting the Foundation

Elizabeth Speakman, EdD, RN, CDE, FNAP, ANEF

Mary Hanson-Zalot, EdD, MSN, RN, AOCN, CNE

Whereas interprofessional team-based care has advanced in Canada, the United Kingdom, and Australia, it remains isolated in the United States. Political and social events such as the passing of the Patient Protection and Affordable Care Act (2010), and the resurgence of the value of high-functioning teams, created a renewed interest in the interprofessional education (IPE) and collaborative practice (CP) movement. But the resurgence for the most part focused on creating interprofessional learning opportunities for students. The dichotomy is that "today's students who graduate from well-intended, well-accredited institutions are simply unprepared for the practice environments in which they will work (Speakman & Arenson, 2015, p. 3). Therefore, if students do not engage in collaborative clinical experiences, or do not witness collaboration among health professionals in practice, their interprofessional classroom learning experiences are for naught. Furthermore, Cox and Naylor (2013) warn that unless we can link team-based care to improved patient outcomes, then providing interprofessional care will fall short of meeting the healthcare needs of patients and communities in the 21st century.

THE INTERPROFESSIONAL EDUCATION AND COLLABORATIVE PRACTICE MOVEMENT AND THE HISTORY OF NURSING

Social, political, economic, and environmental factors have always prominently influenced nursing practice and nursing education. Therefore, when examining the value of IPE and CP in nursing education, it is important to place it within the historical context of education and practice. Box 1.1 describes examples of significant historical events that serve as testimony to the profession's ability to adapt to meet the needs of society.

Today's nurses work in the social-political-economic era of technology-rich environments, where high-tech, high-acuity patient care is delivered. Contemporary healthcare reform measures work to keep people out of hospital settings and support "age in place" living by managing chronicity in the community and a mandated healthcare

---

BOX 1.1

Historical Examples of How Nursing Has Met Society's Needs

- Florence Nightingale using her political influence to get permission from the British Secretary of War to travel to Crimea
- Volunteer "nurses" leaving their families during the Civil War, forever changing public opinion about women's role in healthcare
- Nursing visionaries working with Susan B. Anthony on the suffrage, abolition, and human rights movement of the 19th century
- Focusing on community-based healthcare with the establishment of the Henry Street Settlement by Lillian Wald and Mary Brewster, who delivered home nursing care to New York's immigrant population
- Establishing nursing associations like the American Nurses Association (ANA) and the National League for Nursing (NLN), and subsequent registration and licensure through the Nurse Practice Act
- The landmark 1923 Goldmark report, which recommended that the focus of schools of nursing should be on education, not on patient care, and moved it to the university setting
- Embedding nursing programs in community and junior colleges in response to the nursing shortage post WWII, giving men (many returning GIs) and married women the ability to become registered nurses
- Developing the role of the nurse practitioner to work with underserved populations, and the use of formalized research to create evidence-based practice

---

Source: Egenes, K. J. (2009). History of nursing. In G. Roux & J. A. Halstead (Eds.), *Issues and trends in nursing: Essential knowledge for today and tomorrow* (pp. 1–26). Burlington, MA: Jones & Bartlett.

---

act that promises to insure a record number of Americans. As the nursing profession grapples to accommodate this current healthcare delivery system, it has become even more relevant for nurses to collaborate with other healthcare professionals. Therefore, the resurgence of interprofessional practice is both timely and appropriate, but "the health and education systems must work together to coordinate health workforce strategies. If health workforce planning and policymaking are integrated, interprofessional education and collaborative practice can be fully supported" (World Health Organization [WHO], 2010, p. 10). Considering that nursing and nursing education are inextricably connected, nurse educators have to create IPE and CP learning opportunities for students to prepare them to practice in today's healthcare delivery systems.

SIGNIFICANCE OF INTERPROFESSIONAL EDUCATION'S IMPACT ON NURSING PRACTICE

Interestingly, nurses have always worked in interprofessional teams. Extracting nursing from the team is simply impossible; however, somewhere between the high technology and super specialty era, the act of collaboration and integration of teams from multiple professions has weaned away. Healthcare rendered by professionals working in silos is often completely devoid of critical communication and team approaches that if used favor positive patient outcomes. This phenomenon has led to a fragmented healthcare environment that has the greatest potential and risk for errors (Institute of Medicine [IOM], 1972, 1999, 2001, 2003).

It has already been established that nursing and nursing education have a long history of being able to respond to societal needs. Yet this "call to action" is quite different. The ability to create IPE and CP learning experiences for nursing students requires concerted curriculum planning with program plans of study outside of nursing. Even if faculty from multiple disciplines are willing to collaborate, the logistics of assimilating classroom and clinical schedules can be a great obstacle.

Nonetheless, interprofessional teaching and learning are invaluable activities for students matriculated into nursing education programs. Without a doubt, the importance of interprofessional collaboration has been increasingly recognized in the practice, research, and health policy realms (Cohen, 2015). Hence, the inextricable relationship of IPE to the practice setting for student nurses. Additionally, one of the competencies from the Quality and Safety Education for Nurses (QSEN) framework recommends that student nurses learn to engage in open communication and practice collaborative skills with other members of the healthcare team. By doing so, mutual respect is fostered, leading to shared decision making on issues related to patient-centered care (QSEN Institute, 2014). For caregivers to provide safe, high-quality care to patients or communities, there must be appreciation for the complexity of problems presented and the array of options or solutions available to resolve them. The range of alternative solutions to address individual or larger community problems can only be fully recognized if consideration is given to the contributions of all healthcare team members. Introducing IPE early in the professional curricula offers value to students in two ways. The first benefit instills in students the importance of considering others' contributions to healthcare, whereas the second is derived from creating opportunities for learners to hone their communication skills for use with patients, their families, and professional team members.

The heart of interprofessional care is collaboration among members of the healthcare team with the expectation that the patient will be the center of that team and able to express his or her individual needs, priorities, and preferences for healthcare. Ideally, these needs are met through the creation of an interprofessional plan of care. To get to the point of developing, executing, and evaluating such a plan, three fundamental concepts must be established. First, student members of the team must come to know what each discipline contributes to the care of the patient based on its role. Second, students must embrace the notion that the ability to communicate, which is pivotal to interprofessional work, and learning to collaborate are skills that will serve them well throughout their professional and personal lives. Third, students must recognize the tangible and intangible influences of culture derived from the academic environment, their selected discipline, and the practice setting. Awareness of these three principles will assist faculty in designing and focusing learning opportunities for students across the levels in nursing.

HEALTHCARE TEAM MEMBER CONTRIBUTION

As mentioned previously, the United States has lagged behind the international community in integrating IPE and CP in health professions education. However, in 2011, a framework for integrating IPE and CP in the United States was published by the Interprofessional Education Collaborative (IPEC) Expert Panel, and in Chapter 2 the IPEC Core Competencies are described in greater detail. One of the core competencies of interprofessional CP is to understand the specific roles and responsibilities undertaken by each member of the healthcare team (Interprofessional Education Collaborative [IPEC] Expert Panel, 2011). Activities designed to bring students together from a variety of disciplines should be intentional and goal directed. Providing structure for these sessions is critical for students to begin learning with and about each other—a tenet of the 2010 World Health Organization (WHO) report. One of the most direct ways of providing a session about roles and responsibilities is through implementation of an active learning strategy, such as the use of a case study. This method allows students to practice critical thinking skills and familiarizes them with the work of professional students from other disciplines. Allowing time for students to converse in teams can be highly beneficial to their learning. Cox and Naylor (2013) note that the use of team scenario building can be an important learning opportunity, especially when there are educational and practice resource constraints.

Creating opportunities for students to work together and learn each other's role creates positive relationships. Dutton, Roberts, and Bednar (2010) posit that building social relationships strengthens an employee's work-related identity. Furthermore, Flicek (2012) noted that the lack of coeducational experiences where health professionals understood each other's roles affected their ability to communicate when they copracticed.

Communication/Collaboration Skills

IPE activities embedded into the didactic and clinical curriculum, as well as those spontaneous opportunities that arise through student activities on campus, serve as foundational platforms to develop communication abilities. Clinical education comprises a large segment of the curriculum for prelicensure student nurses, and it is in this setting that they practice the skills of communication, collaboration, and problem solving during interactions with patients, professional nursing staff, clinical faculty, and other members of the healthcare team. The delivery of quality patient care requires that health professionals feel comfortable and communicate effectively with one another. The Joint Commission (2012) concluded that 80 percent of serious medical errors are the result of miscommunication between caregivers during the handoff period.

Communication skills allow students and practitioners to discern the nature of patient problems and clarify the goals and priorities of the patient. This knowledge is crucial to the development of clinical reasoning ability. Clinical reasoning may be defined as "the application of knowledge and clinical experience towards a clinical presentation to derive a solution" (Noll, Key, & Jensen, 2001, p. 41). Benner, Sutphen, Leonard, and Day (2010) describe clinical reasoning as "the ability to reason about a clinical situation as it unfolds, as well as about patient and family concerns and context" (p. 46). Strength in clinical reasoning ability may be related to patient outcomes (Kuiper, 2013). Alfaro-LeFevre (2012) asserts that the nursing process, with its five-step model of assessment, diagnosis, planning, implementation, and evaluation, is the foundation of clinical reasoning. This process is enhanced by considering those elements of care best met by the various healthcare team members who interact with the patient. Students who practice collaboration while in school ultimately become practitioners who will collaborate once graduated.

The role of faculty is not to appeal to every student's learning preference, or to follow traditional lock-step methods of teaching (Brookfield, 1986). Benner et al. (2010) suggest that faculty move away from teaching practices that do not incorporate active engagement in learning. They assert that nursing classes should stimulate powerful learning, with each class designed to help students develop their "clinical imagination" (p. 79). Inclusion of team members from other disciplines in creative and active processes promotes added value to the learning experiences crafted. Communication between team members breaks down the traditional silos that have existed historically in health professions education. "Although most health professionals and educators agree that the use of team approaches to learning and solving healthcare problems is the best way to teach, the clinical and educational environment frequently remains prohibitive to team training and tends to support silo learning and practice" (Speakman & Arenson, 2015, p. 3).

The Influence of Culture

Culture may be defined as "what a group learns over a period of time as that group solves its problems of survival in an external environment and its problems of internal integration" (Schein, 1990, p. 111). Students in schools of nursing interface with culture at multiple levels. The culture of the school, the culture of the profession they have chosen, and the culture of the institution where they engage in clinical learning all need to be considered in designing student learning experiences. The external environment that students are subject to already exists. Where there is opportunity to move as a group is through internal integration as offered by Schein (1990). By introducing IPE early, students become aware of some of the cultural attributes ascribed to other professions as well as their own, thus facilitating their understanding of each other's roles. Additionally, students can be empowered to *create* culture and move this system of values and priorities into the practice realm upon graduation. Students who actively participate in these new models of interaction and thinking are more apt to embrace these tendencies as graduate practitioners. Typically, it is not what the teacher does in the teaching-learning process, but what the student does that is learned (Williams & Nations, 1978). However, the unintended consequences of preparing students in an educational system designed to match the "old" healthcare system is that it is void of the opportunity to practice teamwork skills and shared decision making (Speakman & Arenson, 2015). Nursing education has a history of reconceptualizing how to prepare nurses for practice settings. The multiple entry paths, the addition of evidence-based practice and community health nursing, and advanced practice certifications and degrees are examples of how the profession responded to societal healthcare needs. Creating an educational environment that includes IPE and CP is today's societal need that will prepare nurses to engage in team-based patient-centered care.

Modeled Behavior

Considering the assertion of Bandura (1977) that individuals adopt a modeled behavior if that behavior is similar to them and has admired status, it is conceivable that students who are only taught by a solo practitioner are destined to repeat that behavior whether that behavior is correct or not. In fact, hierarchies too often prohibit learning the roles and responsibilities, expertise, opinions, and suggestions of other professions (Speakman & Arenson, 2015). For students to engage in team-based care, they must be exposed to diverse thoughts and methods. It has already been established that there is a correlation between understanding another health professional's role, effective communication, and patient outcomes (IPEC Expert Panel, 2011). Although it might be correct to state that many practitioners learn this correlation when they are in practice, the question then is how might patient outcomes have been improved if this were taught when the practitioner was a student? It is logical to conclude that students exposed to team training and who observe team-based care while learning will model these positive behaviors at the onset of their practice.

IMPLICATIONS OF INTERPROFESSIONAL EDUCATION AND COLLABORATIVE PRACTICE ON NURSING EDUCATION

Many nurse educators agree that nursing students should be experiencing interprofessional learning opportunities and CP clinical opportunities; however, they continue to be challenged by the complexity of implementation. The logistics of integration, such as competing schedules, often impede creating true IPE opportunities. How then can IPE be measurable and sufficient to impact the delivery of care? Does it take a true immersion, or does exposure to multiple opportunities, regardless of length, have an impact on culture and behavior?

Transformative learning occurs when adults experience frames of references that define their life world (Mezirow, 1997). Therefore, each interprofessional experience has an impact that can change a student's behavior and learning. The implication is simply that introducing IPE can be done in a variety of ways and through a variety of methods. Although it might be correct to hope that more is better, the fact remains that getting students to interact with other members of the healthcare team early in their program will allow them to envision diversity of thought surrounding patient care approaches. It has already been established that today's healthcare delivery systems' idiosyncrasies can best be managed by the collective wisdom of a team of health professionals. This changing landscape of the healthcare delivery system, as well as the changes to come in the future as technology intersects patient care, will require the nurse to be an effective member and leader of the healthcare delivery team. Although the concepts of teamwork can be taught in the silo of the nursing curriculum, they cannot be effectively practiced in nursing alone. Nurses, as well as all students in the health professions, need time to practice together and engage in group thinking and problem solving if they are going to engage in those behaviors as practicing clinicians.

How Can Interprofessional Education Be Implemented in Nursing Curricula?

It appears that some nursing programs seem to have an advantage in implementing IPE and CP learning opportunities because of affiliations; however, that is actually not the case. There are many ways in which nursing curricula can implement team training and the concepts of patient-centered care and effective communication. Remember that not every student nor every graduate will have the same IPE and CP experience. Furthermore, each type of nursing program should recognize that all levels of the nursing profession are central to the delivery of care and valuable members of the healthcare delivery team. Box 1.2 outlines exemplars of how IPE and CP learning opportunities may be incorporated into the nursing curriculum. Specific IPE and CP learning activities are found in detail in each subsequent chapter of this book and in the IPE toolkit on the National League for Nursing website (Speakman, Tagliareni, Sherburne, & Sicks, 2016).

BOX 1.2

Exemplars for Interprofessional Education and Collaborative Practice Opportunities for Nursing Programs

A Classroom (Didactic) IPE Learning Exemplar

1. Invite students and faculty representatives from programs outside of nursing to join your class. (*Note:* Students do not have to be enrolled in a health professions program plan of study.)
2. Divide students into groups, making sure that each group includes representation from each program.
3. Have each student group work on a team-training skill activity, such as follows:
   a. Lifeboat challenge (www.createdebate.com)
   b. Marshmallow challenge (www.leadershipchallenge.com)
   c. Lego™ building (www.quickteambuildingactivities.com)
4. As a faculty team, debrief with students about how they worked in a team:
   a. Did anyone lead the team?
   b. Did the entire team make decisions?
   c. Did they encounter any obstacles? If so, how did they resolve the issue(s)?
   d. What communication skills did they use?
   e. How would they apply what they learned about teamwork and communication skills to their respective profession?

A Simulation IPE and CP Learning Exemplar

1. Invite students and faculty representatives from programs outside of nursing to join your class. (*Note:* Students do not have to be enrolled in a health professions program plan of study.)
2. Divide students into groups, making sure that each group includes representation from each program.
3. Build a simulation scenario based on the type of student population in attendance:
   a. For nursing and other allied health professions, the simulation can be a medical emergency, ensuring that the complexity correlates to the year in the program (sirc.nln.org) or a year in training.
   b. For nursing and non–allied health students, the simulation can be a disaster with or without minor injuries, like an active shooter (www.calhospitalprepare.org).
4. As a faculty team, debrief with students about how they worked in a team:
   a. Did anyone lead the team?
   b. Did the entire team make decisions?
   c. Did they encounter any obstacles? If so, how did they resolve the issue(s)?
   d. What communication skills did they use?
   e. How would they apply what they learned about teamwork and communication skills to their respective profession?

Clinical (Experiential) CP Exemplars

1. Find opportunities to discuss both pre- and or postconference the tenets of team-based patient-centered care. Be sure to use examples.
2. Multiple health professionals round with their respective students. Have the clinical faculty request that the nursing student caring for the patient joins the team. Debrief the experience postconference.
3. Find opportunities in the clinical setting for students to engage with other healthcare students on the unit. For example, ask pharmacy students to work with nursing students on a "teach-back" activity (www.teachbacktraining.org). Debrief the experience postconference.

SETTING THE FOUNDATION FOR INTERPROFESSIONAL EDUCATION AND COLLABORATIVE PRACTICE IN NURSING EDUCATION

As noted in this chapter and throughout the following chapters, creating and implementing IPE and CP requires a concerted effort. First and foremost is the necessity to understand IPE and CP. Consider the *why, who, what,* and *where* framework.

The *Why*

Examine the literature that supports IPE and CP. The landmark Institute of Medicine (IOM) reports (IOM, 1972, 1999, 2001, 2003) explore the impact of team-based patient-centered care on quality and safety. Subsequent IPE and CP literature explores why the healthcare environment needs the collective wisdom of a team. In essence, we must be able to meet today's societal health needs in a technology-rich environment caring for high-acuity patients in tertiary care centers, as well as chronically ill patients in outpatient or community centers. Finally, the 2010 IOM *Future of Nursing* report recommends that nurses have an integral role as valuable members of the team in providing team-based care (IOM, 2010).

The *Who*

The IPE and CP literature over the past three decades clearly demonstrates the importance of collaboration and team-based care. As discussed previously, the WHO advises that healthcare workforce planning is the coordination of the healthcare system and healthcare education (WHO, 2010). As a result of this assertion and similar published documents, most health profession accrediting agencies are now requiring students to learn and practice in interprofessional teams.

The *What*

As previously noted in this chapter, and as will be described in subsequent chapters, IPE and CP learning opportunities can be accomplished in a variety of ways. The underlining key is to have students engaged with one another in meaningful ways that best assist them to meet the IPEC Core Competencies. Whether students are engaged with only one other profession or a multitude of professions, whether with other health profession students or not, bringing students together to develop skills in communication, teamwork, or problem solving will prepare them to work in the contemporary healthcare delivery system.

The *Where*

IPE and CP learning experiences can occur in myriad places within the nursing curriculum and should include opportunities in the classroom, clinical environment, and simulation laboratory. To ensure that students can meet the IPEC Core Competencies, as noted in detail in Chapter 2, a systematic plan of activities using the core competencies as the header is suggested. Refer to Table 1.1 for a schematic plan.

TABLE 1.1			
Systematic Plan of Interprofessional Education and Collaborative Practice Activities and IPEC Core Competencies			
	Interprofessional Team and Teamwork	Interprofessional Communication Practices	Values and Ethics for Interprofessional Practice	Roles and Responsibilities for CP
Classroom			
Clinical			
Simulation			

Note: Some IPE and CP activities may be able to meet more than one IPEC Core Competency.

CONCLUSION

The benefit derived from IPE is that it allows and opportunity for students from a variety of backgrounds and disciplines to communicate with each other. Ultimately, combined effort and communication among team members will provide for safe and effective patient-centered care. Effective and better patient outcomes occur when collaborative teams complement one another and work together (Meleis, 2016). As a foundation of this book, this chapter explores and supports how the nursing profession exercises its integral role in the delivery of healthcare in the 21st century. It also challenges nursing education leaders to recognize that nurses will not be able to engage in team-based patient-centered care if they are not given opportunities to practice the skills in the learning environment. This chapter acknowledges the challenges associated with implementing IPE and CP activities, and in this and subsequent chapters, the reader is offered exemplars of meaningful IPE and CP learning opportunities. "Effective teamwork requires a transformation of how health professionals are educated" (Meleis, 2016, p. 107).

References

Alfaro-LeFevre, R. (2012). Nursing process and clinical reasoning. *Nursing Education Perspectives, 33*(1), 7.

Bandura, A. (1977). Self-efficacy: Toward a unifying theory of behavioral change. *Psychological Review, 84*(2), 191–215.

Benner, P., Sutphen, M., Leonard, V., & Day, L. (2010). *Educating nurses: A call for radical transformation.* San Francisco: Carnegie/Jossey-Bass.

Brookfield, S. D. (1986). *Understanding and facilitating adult learning.* San Francisco: Jossey-Bass.

Cohen, S. S. (2015). Interprofessional and interdisciplinary collaboration: Moving forward. *Policy, Politics, and*

Nursing Practice, 14(3–4), 115–116. doi:10.1177/1527154414533616.

Cox, M., & Naylor, M. (2013). *Transforming patient care: Aligning interprofessional education with clinical practice redesign.* New York: Josiah Macy Jr. Foundation.

Dutton, J. E., Roberts, L. M., & Bednar, J. (2010). Pathways for positive identity construction at work: Four types of positive identity and the building of social resources. *Academy of Management Review, 35*(2), 265–293.

Egenes, K. J. (2009). History of nursing. In G. Roux & J. A. Halstead (Eds.), *Issues and trends in nursing: Essential knowledge for today and tomorrow* (pp. 1–26). Burlington, MA: Jones & Bartlett.

Flicek, C. L. (2012). Communication: A dynamic between nurses and physicians. *Medsurg Nursing, 21*(6), 385–387.

Institute of Medicine. (1972). *Educating a healthcare team: Report of the conference.* Washington, DC: National Academy of Sciences.

Institute of Medicine. (1999). *To err is human: Building a safer health care system.* Washington, DC: National Academies Press.

Institute of Medicine. (2001). *Crossing the quality chasm: A new health system for the 21st century.* Washington, DC: National Academies Press.

Institute of Medicine. (2003). *A bridge to quality.* Washington, DC: National Academies Press.

Institute of Medicine. (2010). *The future of nursing: Leading change, advancing health.* Washington, DC: National Academies Press.

Interprofessional Education Collaborative Expert Panel. (2011). *Core competencies for interprofessional collaborative practice: Report of an expert panel.* Washington, DC: Interprofessional Education Collaborative.

Joint Commission on Accreditation of Healthcare Organizations. (2012). Joint Commission Center for transforming healthcare releases targeted solutions tool for hand-off communications. *Joint Commision Perspectives, 32*(8), 1–2.

Retrieved from http://www.jointcommission.org/assets/1/6/tst_hoc_persp_08_12.pdf

Kuiper, R. A. (2013). Integration of innovative clinical reasoning pedagogies into a baccalaureate nursing curriculum. *Creative Nursing, 19*(3), 128–139. doi:10.1891/10784535.19.3.128

Meleis, A. I. (2016). Interprofessional education: A summary of reports and barriers to recommendations. *Journal of Nursing Scholarship, 48*(1), 106–112.

Mezirow, J. (1997). Transformative learning: Theory to practice. *New Directions for Adult and Continuing Education, 74*, 5–12. doi: 10.1002/ace.7401

Noll, E., Key, A., & Jensen, G. (2001). Clinical reasoning of an experienced physiotherapist: Insight into clinical decision making regarding low back pain. *Physiotherapy Research International, 6*, 40–51. doi:10.1002/pri.212

Patient Protection and Affordable Care Act. (2010). 42 U.S.C. § 18001 et seq.

QSEN Institute. (2014). Competencies. Retrieved June 5, 2016, from http://qsen.org/competencies/

Schein, E. H. (1990). Organizational culture. *American Psychologist, 45*(2), 109–119.

Speakman, E., & Arenson, C. (2015). Going back to the future: What is all the buzz about interprofessional education and collaborative practice? *Nurse Educator, 41*(3), 3–4.

Speakman, E., Tagliareni, E., Sherburne, A., & Sicks, S. (2016). *Guide to effective interprofessional education experiences in nursing education.* Washington, DC: National League for Nursing.

Williams, P. E., & Nations, L. B. (1978). The teaching-learning process. In *Curriculum development and its implementation through a conceptual framework* (pp. 47–59). New York: National League for Nursing.

World Health Organization. (2010). *Framework for action on interprofessional education and collaborative practice.* Geneva, Switzerland: Author. Available at http://apps.who.int/iris/bitstream/10665/70185/1/WHO_HRH_HPN_10.3_eng.pdf

2

Core Competencies and the Kirkpatrick Model: A Framework for Interprofessional Education and Collaborative Practice

Christine Arenson, MD

WHY INTERPROFESSIONAL EDUCATION, AND WHY COMPETENCIES?

The Institute of Medicine (IOM) landmark *Future of Nursing* (2011) report highlighted the need for interprofessional practice and teamwork among members of the healthcare team. Concomitant is the steadfast notion that today's healthcare must focus on the delivery of safe, quality, patient-centered care.

In 1972, the IOM first articulated the need for interprofessional education for all health professionals (Institute of Medicine [IOM], 1972). Interprofessional education and collaboration has continued to be identified as a cornerstone strategy to deliver high-quality, safe, effective, efficient, patient-centered, team-based care (IOM, 2003). Over the years, many national and international organizations have reaffirmed the need for interprofessional education, including the Agency for Healthcare Research and Quality (AHRQ), Health Resources and Services Administration (HRSA), the Josiah Macy Jr. Foundation, Pew Commission, Robert Wood Johnson Foundation (RWJF), and the World Health Organization (WHO) (American Interprofessional Health Collaborative, 2011; Hopkins, 2010).

Competency-based assessment of nursing education has been advocated since at least the 1970s (Del Bueno, 1978) and is now widely accepted in nursing education practice (National League for Nursing, 2012, 2015). With adoption of the Next Accreditation System for graduate medical education in the United States (Nasca, Philibert, Brigham, & Flynn, 2012), medicine as a discipline officially adopted competency-based evaluation as the ideal for certifying clinicians. Leaders in the interprofessional education movement have stressed the need for competency-based assessment of collaborative practice skills for nearly two decades (Barr, 1998).

INTERPROFESSIONAL EDUCATION AND COLLABORATIVE PRACTICE COMPETENCIES AROUND THE GLOBE

The movement toward competency-based assessment of health professions education generally, coupled with specific discussion within the interprofessional education and collaborative practice communities, has led to the development of a variety of interprofessional education competency frameworks. Among the first in the United States were a series of specialty-specific competencies, exemplified by the document *Multidisciplinary Competencies in the Care of Older Adults at the Completion of the Entry-Level Health Professional Degree* (Partnership for Health in Aging, 2008). This document was created using a Delphi methodology, soliciting input from a variety of educators from across the fields of geriatrics and gerontology, and sought to improve the readiness of new health professionals to care for the complex issues of aging.

These topic-focused competencies have been followed by the development of competencies to prepare collaborative practice–ready practitioners across any point in the care continuum and regardless of population served. *Framework for Action on Interprofessional Education and Collaborative Practice* (Hopkins, 2010) set an international standard for the key domains and issues needed for effective collaborative practice. National competency frameworks in Canada (Canadian Interprofessional Health Collaborative, 2010) and the United States (Interprofessional Education Collaborative Practice [IPEC] Expert Panel, 2011) identify many overlapping themes and competencies, tailored for the specific issues, challenges, and resources of their national healthcare and education systems.

The U.S. competencies (IPEC Expert Panel, 2011) place collaborative practice within the context of a patient- and family-centered care system with a community and population orientation, consistent with ongoing redesign of the U.S. healthcare system. The Expert Panel identifies four domains of competency, including:

> Interprofessional Teamwork and Team-Based Practice

> Interprofessional Communication Practices

> Values/Ethics for Interprofessional Practice

> Roles and Responsibilities for Collaborative Practice

Several specific, behaviorally based competencies are defined under each domain, such as Values and Ethics 2: Respect the dignity and privacy of patients while maintaining confidentiality in the delivery of team-based care.

These competency frameworks have served to clarify and codify universal themes of core behaviors that support collaborative practice and person-centered care. Despite highly variable contexts of care and resources, fundamentals translate remarkably well across national boundaries. Increasingly, U.S. accrediting bodies are identifying implementation of the Core Competencies for Interprofessional Collaborative Practice (IPEC Expert Panel, 2011) as an expectation of health professions education programs in nursing, medicine, physical therapy, occupational therapy, and pharmacy, among others.

IMPACT OF COMPETENCIES ON INTERPROFESSIONAL EDUCATION AND COLLABORATIVE PRACTICE

Although interprofessional education has been widely embraced as a core strategy to prepare current and future healthcare providers, widespread adoption remains limited by perceived and actual barriers at the institutional, program, faculty, and student levels. In addition, the evidence from systematic reviews indicate that interprofessional education programs vary in terms of content, duration, and professional participation and that studies evaluating this form of education are of variable quality, arguing for a more systematic approach to implementing team-based education and care (Reeves, Goldman, Burton, & Sawatsky-Girling, 2010). It is imperative to dissect the interprofessional education curriculum, as well as what students are taking away from their interprofessional experiences, yet it is also imperative to examine if training institutions offering interprofessional education programs are teaching the "best practices" of collaborative care. Although numerous institutions have implemented various courses and programs designed to provide students in the health professions with learning opportunities steeped in interprofessional education (Nisbet, Hendry, Rolls, & Field, 2008; Blue, Zoller, Stratton, Elam, & Gilbert, 2010; Curran, Sharpe, Flynn, & Button, 2010), there has been little effort to investigate if the principles of these programs are indeed the fundamental tenets of collaborative practice that are employed in the professional field.

Questions also remain related to the infrastructure required to develop, implement, evaluate, and sustain effective interprofessional education in nursing, medicine, and other health professional programs. For example, what are the optimum strategies to teach core collaborative practice competencies in an effective interprofessional environment in a classroom, simulation/laboratory, or clinical setting? Although a clear set of competencies has been identified, these have not yet been fully operationalized to support implementation. Team-based care has been effectively argued to be essential for safe, patient-centered, healthcare delivery (Lurie, Schultz, & Lamanna, 2011; Leonard & Frankel, 2011). However, little is known regarding how aspects of the overarching culture of a practice (at the meso- and macro levels) impact how and in what manner individuals form and behave as a "team" (micro level)—and how this macro-micro interaction fosters or hinders patient and/or provider well-being.

Therefore, if team-based care is a fundamental element of positive healthcare delivery, then understanding the logistical elements of team building and team maintenance in the healthcare setting is paramount to fostering a favorable and sustainable transformation experience for collaborative practice. For practice teams to function effectively and efficiently, the team must have the proper structure, roles must be clearly identified, coordinating mechanisms must be in place, and communication lines must be effective among providers and patients (Leonard & Frankel, 2011). Effective team structure and process allow the members of the team to "practice at the top of their license." Inefficiencies resulting from members spending time doing tasks for which other team members are better prepared and/or coordination errors are eliminated. Effective team practices and interprofessional collaboration should result in enhanced patient care. Other questions include the following: What is the impact of team-based care on patients, families, and community health? What are the characteristics of learning and clinical environments that result in high-quality learning and care? And how does faculty participation in interprofessional education affect teaching productivity? The report by the Interprofessional Collaborative Practice (IPEC) Expert Panel (2011) also suggested additional challenges at the institutional level, including a lack of institutional collaborators and faculty development issues.

Further, there are conflicting anecdotal reports that faculty workload increases with interprofessional education, institutional and professional accreditation issues can hamper adoption, and financial and nonfinancial rewards are not in place to sustain faculty participation. Thistlewaite et al. (2014) argue effectively for adopting common language, strengthening academic and practice partnerships, and improving assessment of collaborative practice competencies to ensure that future practitioners are entering practice well prepared for successful collaborations and team-based care.

Barriers can be overcome by (a) operationalizing the competencies required for interprofessional education in classroom, simulation/laboratory, and clinical settings; (b) assessing infrastructure requirements for implementing and sustaining interprofessional education; (c) determining best practices that support interprofessional education and collaborative practice; and (d) addressing outcomes of interprofessional approaches (Thistlewaite et al., 2014). A recent review of 83 studies of interprofessional education interventions continues to find inconsistencies in design, implementation, and evaluation of interprofessional education, which continue to hamper the ability of educators to develop and students to achieve interprofessional collaborative learning (Abu-Rish et al., 2012).

IMPLICATIONS FOR EVALUATION OF INTERPROFESSIONAL EDUCATION AND COLLABORATIVE PRACTICE INITIATIVES

International leaders in interprofessional education and assessment of team learning continue to call for the need to employ pedagogically sound theoretical frameworks to the design, delivery, and assessment of interprofessional education to promote collaborative practice (Barr, 2013; Reeves & Hean, 2013; Thistlewaite, 2012). Importantly, recent conferences and white papers have increasingly emphasized the need to link interprofessional education with practice redesign that supports collaborative practice and that is both patient- and family-centered (CFAR, Inc., Tomasik, & Fleming, 2015; IOM, 2013, 2015; Cox & Naylor, 2013).

Linking improved patient- or population-level health outcomes to educational interventions has proved elusive, although education programs are increasingly expected to hold themselves to this standard.

THE KIRKPATRICK MODEL AS AN EXEMPLAR EVALUATION FRAMEWORK FOR INTERPROFESSIONAL EDUCATION AND COLLABORATIVE PRACTICE INITIATIVES

The Kirkpatrick model of educational program evaluation (Kirkpatrick, 1979; Kaufman, Keller, & Watkins, 1995) defines a four-level framework:

> *Level 1:* Reaction (how learners feel about instruction)

> *Level 2:* Learning (learner performance on written tests)

> *Level 3:* Behavior (extent to which learners implement, or transfer, what they learned in class, i.e., performance on behaviorally based competency assessments)

> *Level 4:* Results (organizational benefits, i.e., improvements in individual patient or population health outcomes, or improved metrics of work performance and satisfaction among professional team members)

The original Kirkpatrick model asserted positive causal relationships from learner reactions to learning to behavior to results. An evaluation of three decades of evidence from application of the Kirkpatrick model (Alliger & Janak, 1989) questioned the linear causal links but supported the four levels of training and suggested a recursive model among learning, behavior, and results. To assess interprofessional education, consider all four levels by contemplating trainees' reactions via engagement in and response to inter-professional collaboration. Interprofessional learning entails the development of beliefs, value, and understanding across professions. The behavioral manifestation of learning is the development during training and the application in the collaborative practice work environment of collaboration and communication skills and habits, and the adoption of appropriate roles vis-a-vis one's own profession and the professions of others. Collabo-rative practice teams that demonstrate effective behaviors should demonstrate results including enhanced patient, family, and community engagement; improved healthcare metrics; better health of patients and populations; and reduced costs of care.

Historically, health professions education programs have addressed Kirkpatrick's Level 1 (Reaction) and Level 2 (Learning) extremely well. However, all too often, time and resource constraints have limited assessment of Level 3 (Behavior) outcomes. Level 4 (Results) outcomes are rarely accessed in standard health professions evalua-tion schema. In fact, historically, health professions education has been largely sepa-rated from the practice environments where transformation to value-based purchasing and consumer-driven healthcare is rapidly redefining what constitutes important results at the level of individual patients, populations, and communities.

CREATING A SYSTEMATIC PLAN OF PROGRAM EVALUATION

Having a systematic plan of program evaluation allows faculty to evaluate curriculum systematically, and with the rigor of research. This permits stakeholders, including accreditors, deans, faculty, students, future employers, and the public, to be confident that the curriculum is thorough (i.e., addresses all identified core competencies) and effective (i.e., learners achieve adequate progress toward competency based on the appropriate educational level and expectations). Finally, it provides a systematic and clear strategy to address the impact of new curriculum on behaviors of learners in clini-cal settings and, with appropriate clinical collaborations, to actually drive assessment into clinical performance and clinical outcomes.

Developing a systematic plan requires faculty to select an evaluation framework, such as the Kirkpatrick model. Additionally, faculty must clearly define and articulate the competencies to be addressed and the expected level of attainment (i.e., familiarity, competency, mastery) to be achieved over the course of the educational program. Ide-ally, a robust systematic plan of evaluation will span the entire professional curriculum— from matriculation to graduation. Within the plan, each educational element (i.e., discrete course or clinical experience) will map to clear competency and mastery objectives.

For instance, a bachelor-level nursing student on the first clinical rotation may be expected to be able to "identify and describe" key elements of the professional roles and responsibilities of the RN, physician, and other health professionals. By graduation, the same nursing student will be expected to demonstrate competency in understanding roles and responsibilities by being able to communicate the RN's roles and responsibili-ties clearly to patients and colleagues (IPEC Competency RR1) and effectively calling on the unique and complementary abilities of all members of the team to optimize patient care (IPEC Competency RR9) (IPEC Expert Panel, 2011).

Ultimately, a systematic plan must be realistic. Faculty and students must have the resources (e.g., time, expertise, and didactic and clinical resources) to accomplish the plan. For instance, the U.S. Core Competencies (IPEC Expert Panel, 2011) identify a total of 38 core competencies for interprofessional collaborative practice across the four domains. Few health professions programs could overlay an additional 38 competencies on top of already packed curricula and strained resources. Further, collaborative practice competencies by definition require collaboration with other professions and professional education programs. Thus, each program and institution must realistically assess its resources and opportunities for the greatest impact on the future success of its graduates. Commonly, institutions are defining a limited set of core competencies for collaborative practice, such as one from each domain or key competencies that address priority institutional concerns. This more manageable set of interprofessional competencies can then be adopted across all health professions programs and monitored by a smaller number of faculty with specific interprofessional education and collaborative practice responsibility.

Once the evaluation framework and specific core competencies have been chosen, the systematic framework can be developed. The plan will be multidimensional, with the competencies intersecting with the Kirkpatrick levels of assessment and tracking longitudinally across each health professions education program. Faculty must be able to readily identify when bachelor-level nursing students are receiving a basic introduction to the core competencies, when they first get to practice the competencies in clinical placements, and when mastery of the competencies will be assessed. A similar approach should be taken for graduate nursing students, medical students, pharmacy students, and other health professions students, in which case faculty must then collaborate across programs to ensure that a nursing student will not be expected to be demonstrating mastery of a competency during an interaction with a pharmacy student who has not yet had a basic introduction to the concept. This requires active and ongoing collaboration among faculty with deep understanding of each health professions curriculum engaged in institutional interprofessional education efforts.

DEMONSTRATING RESULTS: PARTNERING WITH PRACTICE

Although educators have fundamental control of the curriculum and evaluation plan for their students, documentation of Level 4 (Results) outcomes, including both workplace and patient- or population-level clinical outcomes, requires partnership with clinical settings and clinicians. Rigorous evaluation of clinical outcomes requires research skills, personnel, and financial support that will be beyond the scope of many, if not most, educational programs. Nevertheless, creative partnerships between educators and clinicians can yield meaningful assessment of Level 4 outcomes. For instance, an interprofessional activity might engage students from three health professions programs together with a clinician from a shared clinical site to conduct a quality improvement project. The clinic may note improved quality metrics, such as enhanced control of blood pressure among patients who are hypertensive or a higher likelihood of aspirin prescriptions on discharge for patients with acute coronary syndrome as a result of interventions conceived by interprofessional student teams. The patient experience, known to be positively impacted by highly effective collaborative practice teams, may also improve when collaborative interprofessional student teams engage in their care. Educators and clinicians can collaborate using data already collected to meet ongoing quality and patient experience metrics to begin to assess Level 4 outcomes' impact from educational programs.

CORE COMPETENCIES AND THE KIRKPATRICK MODEL: IMPLICATIONS FOR NURSING EDUCATION

The move to incorporate interprofessional education is being driven by an increasing recognition that effective collaborative practice is mandatory to promote safe, effective, and efficient patient-centered care. This movement has been paralleled by a shift toward competency-based assessment of health professions education programs. Interprofessional education provides an ideal opportunity for nursing faculty, in collaboration with other health professions faculty at their own or partner institutions, to drive positive change in our health system by preparing graduates for 21st-century practice.

CONCLUSION

The U.S. healthcare system is rapidly changing to one that is driven by value. Clinicians in hospitals, ambulatory practice, and community-based clinics are rapidly redesigning practice to be successful in new pay-for-performance reimbursement models that aim to promote the Triple Aim: better experience of care, better health outcomes, and lower cost of care. Collaborative practice has been widely accepted as a key support for meeting the Triple Aim (Institute for Healthcare Improvement, 2016).

Organizations across and beyond the United States have recognized that future health professionals must be educated in core competencies of interprofessional teamwork to meet the demands of a rapidly evolving healthcare system.

At the same time, health professions education programs, in nursing as well as other professions, are faced with a variety of economic, pedagogical, and clinical restraints that have made implementing interprofessional education challenging and have limited robust evaluation of educational outcomes. Identification of a structured educational outcomes framework such as the Kirkpatrick model, coupled with adopting a limited set of core interprofessional competencies, will allow educators to create a systematic plan of evaluation that will provide a structured opportunity to map curriculum and assessment and ensure that all students are achieving minimum competencies for future practice. Further, a structured plan of evaluation will facilitate scholarship among nursing faculty and interprofessional educational collaborations across health professions programs.

Finally, it is incumbent on nursing and other health professions faculty to model interprofessional teamwork and collaboration skills for their students and to partner effectively with clinical sites that can provide positive, practical experiences for student teams. "The ability to function on a team, as a team member and as a team leader, and to recognize advances in technology for managing chronic illness in a fundamentally changed healthcare arena is the only way to prepare students" effectively for future practice (Speakman & Arenson, 2015).

References

Abu-Rish, E., Kim, S., Choe, L., Varpio, L., Malik, E., White, A. A., et al. (2012). Current trends in interprofessional education of health sciences students: A literature review. *Journal of Interprofessional Care, 26,* 444–451.

Alliger, G. M., & Janak, E. A. (1989). Kirkpatrick's levels of training criteria: Thirty years later. *Personnel Psychology, 42*(2), 331–342.

American Interprofessional Health Collaborative. (2011, February). *Team-based competencies: Building a shared foundation for education and clinical practice: Conference proceedings.* Washington, DC: Author.

Barr, H. (1998). Competent to collaborate: Towards a competency-based model for interprofessional education. *Journal of Interprofessional Care, 12*(2), 181–187.

Barr, H. (2013). Toward a theoretical framework for interprofessional education. *Journal of Interprofessional Care, 27,* 4–9.

Blue, A. V., Zoller, J., Stratton, T. D., Elam, C. L., & Gilbert, J. (2010). Interprofessional education in US medical schools. *Journal of Interprofessional Care, 24*(2), 204–206.

Canadian Interprofessional Health Collaborative. (2010). *A national interprofessional competency framework.* Vancouver, BC: Author.

CFAR, Inc., Tomasik, J., & Fleming, C. (2015). *Lessons from the field: Promising interprofessional collaboration practices.* Princeton, NJ: Robert Wood Johnson Foundation.

Cox, M., & Naylor, M. (Eds.). (2013, January). *Transforming patient care: Aligning interprofessional education with clinical practice redesign.* Proceedings of a conference sponsored by the Josiah Macy Jr. Foundation, New York.

Curran, V. R., Sharpe, D., Flynn, K., & Button, P. (2010). A longitudinal study of the effect of an interprofessional education curriculum on student satisfaction and attitudes towards interprofessional teamwork and education. *Journal of Interprofessional Care, 24*(1), 41–52.

Del Bueno, D. J. (1978). Competency based education. *Nurse Educator, 3*(3), 10.

Hopkins, D. (Ed.). (2010). *Framework for action on interprofessional education and collaborative practice.* Geneva, Switzerland: World Health Organization.

Institute for Healthcare Improvement. (2016). IHI Triple Aim Initiative. Retrieved June, 1, 2016, from http://www.ihi.org/engage/initiatives/tripleaim/Pages/default.aspx

Institute of Medicine. (1972). *Educating for the health team.* Washington, DC: National Academy of Sciences.

Institute of Medicine. (2003). *Health professions education: A bridge to quality.* Washington, DC: National Academies Press.

Institute of Medicine. (2011). *The future of nursing: Leading change, advancing health.* Washington, DC: National Academies Press.

Institute of Medicine. (2013). *Interprofessional education for collaboration: Learning how to improve health from interprofessional models across the continuum of education to practice.* Washington, DC: National Academies Press.

Institute of Medicine. (2015). *Measuring the impact of interprofessional education on collaborative practice and patient outcomes.* Washington, DC: National Academies Press.

Interprofessional Education Collaborative Expert Panel. (2011). *Core competencies for interprofessional collaborative practice: Report of an expert panel.* Washington, DC: Interprofessional Education Collaborative.

Kaufman, R., Keller, J., & Watkins, R. (1995). What works and what doesn't: Evaluation beyond Kirkpatrick. *Performance + Instruction, 35*(2), 8–12.

Kirkpatrick, D. L. (1979). Techniques for evaluating training programs. *Training and Development Journal, 33*(6), 78–92.

Leonard, M. W, & Frankel, A. S. (2011). Role of effective teamwork and communication in delivering safe, high quality care. *Mount Sinai Journal of Medicine, 78*(6), 820–826.

Lurie, S. J., Schultz, S. H., & Lamanna, G. (2011). Assessing teamwork: A reliable five-question survey. *Family Medicine, 43*(10), 731–734.

Nasca, T. J., Philibert, I., Brigham, T., & Flynn, T. C. (2012). The next GME accreditation system—rationale and benefits. *New England Journal of Medicine, 366*, 1051–1056.

National League for Nursing. (2012). *Outcomes and competencies for graduates of practical/ vocational, diploma, baccalaureate, master's practice, doctorate, and research programs in nursing.* Washington, DC: Author.

National League for Nursing. (2015). *Competencies for nursing education.* Retrieved June 1, 2016, from http://www.nln.org/ professional-development-programs/ competencies-for-nursing-education

Nisbet, G., Hendry, G. D., Rolls, G., & Field, M. J. (2008). Interprofessional learning for prequalification health care students: An outcomes-based evaluation. *Journal of Interprofessional Care, 22*(1), 57–68.

Partnership for Health in Aging. (2008). *Multidisciplinary competencies in the care of older adults at the completion of the entry-level health professional degree.* New York: American Geriatrics Society.

Reeves, S., Goldman, J., Burton, A., & Sawatsky-Girling, B. (2010). Synthesis of systematic review evidence of interprofessional education. *Journal of Allied Health, 39*(3), 198–203.

Reeves, S., & Hean, S. (2013). Why we need theory to help us better understand the nature of interprofessional education, practice and care. *Journal of Interprofessional Care, 27*, 1–3.

Speakman, E., & Arenson, C. (2015). Going back to the future: What is all the buzz about interprofessional education and collaborative practice? *Nurse Educator, 40*(1), 3–4.

Thistlewaite, J. (2012). Interprofessional education: A review of context, learning and the research agenda. *Medical Education, 46*, 58–70.

Thistlewaite, J. E., Forman, D., Matthews, L. R., Rogers, G. D., Steketee, C., & Yassine, T. (2014). Competencies and frameworks in interprofessional education: A comparative analysis. *Academic Medicine, 89*, 869–875.

3

Faculty Development in Interprofessional Education and Interprofessional Collaborative Practice

Mayumi A. Willgerodt, PhD, MPH, RN

Brenda K. Zierler, PhD, RN, FAAN

There is considerable evidence that supports the need for teamwork, effective communication, and interprofessional collaborative practice (IPCP) in healthcare (Reeves, Lewin, Espin, & Zwarenstein, 2010), which traditionally have not been integral components of health professions education. In 2011, the Interprofessional Education Collaborative (IPEC) Expert Panel (2011) identified four domains of competencies as a framework to incorporate interprofessional education (IPE) and collaborative practice (CP) into health professions curriculum. As a result of these established competencies and the resurgence of the value of and need for IPE, many health profession accrediting bodies are now including IPE in their standards. The dichotomy is that faculty (clinician educators, preceptors, academic faculty) are being asked to teach and model CP despite not having been taught the concepts and skills of team science, team communication, or CP. Hence, there is a growing need to provide opportunities to develop faculty to be competent in IPE and IPCP (Anderson, Cox, & Thorpe, 2009). Furthermore, many faculty trained to facilitate learning with students from their own profession may not have been trained to educate interprofessional student teams (Howkins & Bray, 2008; Steinert, 2005; Hall & Zierler, 2015). If students are expected to develop competence in the IPEC domains, faculty need to be supported in developing expertise in teaching and modeling these competencies.

The siloing of health professional education means that most faculty are accustomed to and are experts in teaching uniprofessionally, and nursing education is not immune to this phenomenon. Becoming a competent IPE educator will involve working alongside faculty from other professions to create opportunities for students to learn about, from, and with each other for the purpose of practicing collaboratively (Freeman, Wright, & Lindqvist, 2010; Oandasan & Reeves, 2005). Creating and managing these opportunities can be challenging. Historically, faculty who are used to teaching only their profession's students have potentially disparate teaching pedagogy and styles, and they may only understand their students' learning needs (Buring et al., 2009). Furthermore, teaching interprofessional student teams requires a different approach that accommodates diverse learning styles and perspectives, as well as a sensitivity to the various professional identities. Faculty may report a lack of confidence and feeling of discomfort in their role as interprofessional educators and in their ability to create effective and relevant learning environments for interprofessional groups of students (Bjorke & Haave, 2006; Reeves & Freeth, 2002; Freeman et al., 2010).

The extant literature indicates that faculty development in IPE is an expressed and unmet need among faculty (Anderson et al., 2009; Howkins & Bray, 2008). Contrary to some perceptions, faculty are still committed to participating in faculty development activities because of an appreciation for learning, as well as opportunities for self-improvement and networking with colleagues (Steinert et al., 2010). These individual goals can be leveraged to engage faculty in interprofessional faculty development.

Building IPE competence requires an intentional and systematic faculty development program (Steinert, 2012). Often, faculty participating in IPE activities and events receive "just-in-time" (JIT) training that focuses on the logistics and learning outcomes for the particular event, with little time to discuss the context, rationale for IPE, or challenges in facilitating interprofessional student teams during the activities. Opportunities for discussion among interprofessional faculty or practicing skills, such as providing feedback, facilitating group discussions among interprofessional students, or coteaching, are often missing in JIT faculty trainings. Shrader, Mauldin, Hammad, Mitcham, and Blue (2015) note that faculty often verbalize the need for information about the principles and value-added efforts of IPE and ongoing systematic development opportunities to become proficient in teaching students from multiprofessions.

CREATING FACULTY DEVELOPMENT PROGRAMS IN INTERPROFESSIONAL EDUCATION AND COLLABORATIVE PRACTICE

Steinert (2005) identified three components necessary for effective faculty development programs: engaging faculty, training to facilitate IPE and IPCP, and mentoring for IPE leadership. These can serve as a framework to guide the development and implementation of programs designed to create IPE-competent faculty.

Engaging Faculty

As noted earlier, the majority of faculty have been educated in their own professional silos with little or no opportunity to gain exposure to different professional roles. Additionally, much of what faculty know about teamwork, communication, roles, and values of other health professions has been learned in practice, resulting in differing levels of knowledge, skills, and attitudes related to IPCP (Anderson et al., 2009). Successful IPE depends on engaging faculty across courses, programs, and professions to consistently learn, practice, and model the IPEC Core Competencies.

Content to engage faculty in IPE faculty development programs include definition and rationale for IPE and IPCP, historical and current national and international contexts of IPE, opportunities in and challenges to IPE in educational systems, and exemplar models of CP. Faculty should also learn scopes of practice and responsibilities of the different professions, particularly those with whom they will be teaching and interacting. A lack of knowledge in the roles of other professions impacts the faculty's ability to work and teach effectively together, often perpetuating stereotypes and myths with regard to different professions (Reeves, Lewin, et al., 2010). Interacting and learning content together allows faculty to develop relationships with one another that are grounded in mutual respect and trust, which are essential to support coteaching and collaboration. The development and delivery of activities to engage faculty is an opportunity to be creative and yet purposeful for teaching IPEC Core Competencies. Examples of development activities that engage faculty in IPE content and the process of facilitating IPCP are housed on the National Center for Interprofessional Practice and Education website (https://nexusipe.org).

In addition to learning about the IPEC Core Competencies, engaging faculty by supporting them to cocreate the IPE curriculum or IPE activity (e.g., didactic content, case development, or joint clinical activities) maximizes the success of IPE implementation and sustainability (Willgerodt et al., 2015). Utilizing IPE champions to serve as coaches in creating content, providing advice, and assisting in implementing activities prevents faculty from feeling overburdened, which can negatively impact faculty buy-in (Kreitner & Kinicki, 2008). These types of strategies support and fully engage faculty in understanding, valuing, and integrating IPE into their teaching (Willgerodt et al., 2015).

Training to Facilitate Interprofessional Education and Collaborative Practice

Working with interprofessional groups of students adds another layer of complexity to teaching that otherwise might not exist and therefore requires additional faculty training. Professions often have characteristic ways of teaching, and individual faculty may have established teaching practices, which may impact effective learning among diverse groups of students (Buring et al., 2009). Preparing faculty to teach IPCP should include context setting, process awareness, skills training, and coaching on teaching strategies.

Awareness of one's own professional self is important to understand process-related issues in IPE. Recognizing, addressing, and facilitating implicit and explicit biases, assumptions, and stereotypes in a respectful manner is essential to ensure a positive learning environment for students, particularly since professional socialization occurs during a student's educational experience (Steinert et al., 2006). Educators are often familiar with their own profession's assumptions or biases but may be less familiar with those of other professions. Bringing faculty together to learn about effective interprofessional teaching provides an opportunity for them to learn from each other about the impact of their profession's language, culture, jargon, acronyms, and behaviors on other professions.

Having an understanding of the group process and team dynamics among interprofessional learners is also paramount for successful teaching and learning to occur. For example, faculty need an understanding of different types of interactions that can occur in group processes. Ruiz, Ezer, and Purden (2013) identified three types of interaction when learning is most effective in interprofessional learning contexts:

▸ *Facilitator-controlled interactions* are typically unidirectional, and the facilitator's role is to convey information while students receive the information.

▸ *Facilitator-driven interactions* refer to those where facilitator and students both actively participate in the discussion, yet the content and direction of the dialogue is managed by the facilitator.

▶ *Student-driven interactions* are "owned" by students, and they identify the content and manage the flow and outcomes of the discussion.

In addition, faculty need to possess an understanding of the ways organizational and professional power and hierarchy structures affect these interactions and the resultant group dynamics and processes (Freeth, Hammick, Reeves, Koppel, & Barr, 2005). Faculty also require coaching on how to engage unenthusiastic learners and how to redirect the discussion if one profession dominates the conversation.

Productive learning occurs when students share differing perspectives; however, effective group management is needed when those differences are divided by profession. Group facilitation is a critical skill for which faculty report feeling unprepared, especially with interprofessional groups. Facilitation to promote interaction and effective communication among interprofessional learners is a key teaching strategy (Freeman et al., 2010) and promotes successful learning because students are able to discuss their professions, as well as share perspectives and teach each other about them. Other key skills needed for faculty to be competent in IPE include experience in negotiating or managing differences, facilitating discussions, resolving conflict, providing and accepting feedback, and debriefing or reflecting (Freeth et al., 2005; Steinert, 2005; Howkins & Bray, 2008).

Various instructional approaches that facilitate learning of the IPEC Core Competencies are described throughout this book. However, it is important to note that each of the designs may vary widely depending on context, environment, and experience of the instructors. For example, in the classroom, unfolding cases facilitated by faculty teams allow interprofessional teams of students to cocreate care or treatment plans. Other classroom-based activities might include the use of expert panels of faculty and/or patients discussing a lived experience (e.g., shared decision making or patient-centered care), or they might utilize standardized actors trained to react to students who disclose a team error. In these types of cases, faculty have to be expert at engaging all students, meeting the objectives of the activity, providing feedback, debriefing the case, and coaching the student learners. Approaches to IPE learning outside of the classroom include team-based quality improvement projects, service learning activities in the community, interprofessional journal clubs, and simulated clinical cases in a laboratory setting. All of these approaches should include authentic cases, realistic goals for the activity, and time for students to learn from each other and debrief from the activities. These activities should be facilitated in a manner that promotes shared values and mutual learning.

Approaches to facilitating IPE in clinical settings include interprofessional shadowing (of another profession); observing or participating in briefs, huddles, or interprofessional rounding of patients; or participating in case conferences. These types of activities provide opportunities for students to witness CP and practice teamwork and communication skills. In these environments, the faculty facilitating the debrief or feedback session may be clinical preceptors or other clinician educators, which would require collaboration between the faculty teaching in the classroom with those teaching in practice.

IPE in the clinical setting provides opportunities for students who are in a single discipline and stand-alone program to interact with other learners or practitioners. There are approximately 150 academic health centers in the United States, and students from these institutions are more likely to have an opportunity to participate in IPE activities with other disciplines. However, we know that there are more than 700 nursing programs in the United States, which means that the majority of nursing students are not part of the academic centers with associated schools of medicine, pharmacy, nursing, social work, dentistry, and public health. Ideally, students from stand-alone programs would participate with other professions in the practice environment, shifting IPE in the classroom to IPE in practice (Institute of Medicine [IOM], 2015). Thus, stand-alone nursing programs may have an advantage by not being colocated with other health professions schools, as they are better positioned to employ practice-based meaningful and relevant interprofessional experiences.

Alternatively, many stand-alone nursing schools have found innovative ways to collaborate with other health professions through online or virtual IPE activities. This is also true for online nursing programs (either stand-alone or those housed in academic health centers) that offer distance learning for a majority of the content. Other approaches that support the facilitation of IPE in disparate locations where students are not colocated include the use of online technologies such as asynchronous discussion boards, unfolding case vignettes, and web-based simulations. It is important to note that while convenient, using technology for IPE presents a different set of needed skills. Faculty need to be cognizant that group cohesion and collaboration is delayed with online settings, and possibly reduced altogether. Because one cannot depend on nonverbal cues to gauge learning in this context (Hanna et al., 2013), creating ways that students can demonstrate engagement is essential.

Finally, instructional strategies to facilitate IPE must include appropriate evaluation and assessment that includes both outcome and process measures (Thistlethwaite, Moran, & World Health Organization Study Group on Interprofessional Education and Collaborative Practice, 2010). Faculty who collaborate to develop IPE curricula, activities, or practice opportunities should use a conceptual framework or model described in Chapter 2 to guide the training and the evaluation described in Chapter 10 for assessing learners and evaluating IPE programs.

There is clear evidence that when faculty are taught, coached, and mentored around these skills, not only are they more effective as educators, but students report having more positive and meaningful experiences (Reeves & Freeth, 2002). Further, bringing faculty together to learn how to better meet the learning needs of students may result in a greater appreciation of each other's unique teaching methods and discovery of shared values across professions (Buring et al., 2009; Simmons et al., 2011; Steinert, 2005). Knowing how to promote relevant inquiry in both didactic and clinical settings and engage in active learning strategies such as those described earlier are essential components of faculty development training for IPE.

Mentoring for Interprofessional Education Leadership

Critical to the success and sustainability of IPE and IPCP is the presence of leaders and champions who support, engage in, and actively seek out opportunities for IPE. Faculty development efforts should therefore also incorporate mentoring for IPE leadership. Leadership competencies include facilitating the development of shared goals, becoming an IPE champion, advocating for the flexibility needed for successful IPE, and developing an understanding of organizational structural contexts that impact CP (Bridges, Davidson, Odegard, Maki, & Tomkowiak, 2011; Willgerodt et al., 2015).

BOX 3.1

Faculty Mentoring Exemplar, University of Washington Interprofessional Education Faculty Scholars Program

Eight faculty from three professions were selected to participate in a year-long faculty development program for clinician educators. The IPE faculty scholars then joined the existing physician clinical educators' faculty development program. Whereas the physician clinical educators continued to focus on their individual professional development, the IPE faculty scholars focused on an IPE project as their outcome and had mentors outside of the program who were actively engaged in or leading IPE activities.

Using the faculty development framework of Steinert (2005), the IPE faculty scholars were involved in interprofessional activities, were trained to facilitate IPE through hands-on workshops while pairing them with expert IPE faculty, and continued to be mentored to become leaders in IPE. Of the eight faculty participating in the program, six remained active and are now considered leaders in IPE both at the University of Washington and nationally.

Mentoring could include pairing faculty with experienced IPE educators and facilitators. Identifying and building on the strength of cofacilitating will increase the likelihood that faculty new to IPE will continue to be engaged (Box 3.1).

FACULTY DEVELOPMENT IN INTERPROFESSIONAL EDUCATION CURRICULUM DEVELOPMENT AND IMPLEMENTATION

Interprofessional learning is a process that occurs over time; the IPEC Core Competencies cannot be achieved with one or two stand-alone IPE activities or events. Learning opportunities addressing the competencies need to be woven throughout a curriculum in such a way that makes them visible, explicit, and ongoing. Developing these opportunities requires considerable time and effort, often several times more than what would be required to develop a uniprofessional activity (Buring et al., 2009). Thus, faculty development efforts should also focus on coaching faculty how to develop systematic longitudinal interprofessional curricula that are pedagogically grounded and guided by a framework of interprofessional learning (Willgerodt et al., 2015).

Interprofessional curricula must be guided by pedagogy and adult learning theory (Owen & Schmitt, 2013; Steinert et al., 2006). Appreciative inquiry has been identified as one teaching approach that works well with IPE, as its focus is on creating safe environments that respect individuals and diversity (Dematteo & Reeves, 2011). Other teaching methods that support IPE are communities of learning and practice, as well as problem-based learning (Craddock, O'Halloran, McPherson, Hean, & Hammick, 2013; Sargeant, 2009; Wenger, 1998). A recent Institute of Medicine (IOM) Consensus Committee report entitled *Measuring the Impact of IPE on Collaborative Practice and Patient Outcomes* (IOM, 2015) proposed that a conceptual framework for interprofessional learning should extend across the learning continuum from foundation to graduate to continuing professional development. The report supported the use of adult learning theory and purposeful faculty development, and suggested that successful IPE curricula includes experiential training that moves from the classroom to the practice setting.

Furthermore, rather than creating a stand-alone IPE curriculum, integrating interprofessional learning opportunities into existing courses is a more realistic and sustainable approach to implement IPE, particularly since many programs are already taxed with required courses and clinical experiences, and are challenged to deliver specific content in efficient and cost-effective ways. However, as noted previously, integrating IPE competencies into existing courses requires collaboration among teaching faculty and IPE experts to revise class assignments to incorporate an interprofessional component, to use different approaches to teaching content (e.g., unfolding case-based teaching approaches), and to include other professions or leverage opportunities with other classes to teach common content interprofessionally. In clinical areas, this may involve identifying areas where team-based care or CP is already occurring and having students intentionally participate in those activities. Supporting collaboration across the health professions schools to cocreate IPE activities that can be integrated into courses or curricula is essential for successful implementation and sustainability of IPE. Existing curricula that can be used as resources are available through MedEdPORTAL (https://www.mededportal.org) and other national websites, such as the National Center for Interprofessional Practice and Education (https://nexusipe.org); the University of Washington's Center for Health Sciences Interprofessional Education, Research and Practice (collaborate.uw.edu); the Thomas Jefferson University Center for InterProfessional Education (www.jefferson.edu/university/interprofessional_education.html); and the National League for Nursing Toolkit, *Guide to Effective Interprofessional Education Experiences in Nursing* (www.nln.org).

In addition to understanding effective strategies to develop and implement IPE curricula, faculty also need to be aware of the importance of understanding the different skill sets of interprofessional learners to correctly identify the appropriate leveling of students to be grouped together. Matching the level of students is essential for successful learning, particularly if the case or activity is clinical in nature and requires clinical decision making. The experience is not ideal if, for example, nursing students at the end of their program are grouped with pharmacy or medical students who have yet to enter the clinical arena and are unable to contribute significantly to a discussion involving team-based care. In planning activities, the faculty involved from each profession need to cocreate the IPE activity and determine the appropriate level of students to maximize a successful teamwork experience.

IMPLEMENTATION OF FACULTY DEVELOPMENT PROGRAMS

Hall and Zierler (2015) note that faculty development programs must have clear objectives to ensure efficacy and support ongoing improvements. In addition, faculty development should be led by teams of interprofessional faculty to model teamwork and collaboration. Because of the wide range of faculty who are involved and responsible for IPE, creative approaches to implementing faculty development programs are necessary. The decision to offer real-time, in-person sessions, synchronous or asynchronous online or other virtual methods, or simulations depends on the needs, schedules, and availability of the faculty. Differing learning styles may be accommodated by offering faculty development in a variety of modes, such as seminars, workshops, longitudinal programs, peer coaching, or self-directed learning (Steinert, 2005).

Time is a scarce resource, so faculty development programs must be cognizant of using faculty time well. Providing prework so that faculty are primed and ready to learn when they participate in activities is often most efficient. Prework could include relevant IPE readings (e.g., a Lancet report or an IPEC Core Competencies document) or viewing of primers or videos that lay the foundation for the work that is to occur. Then when faculty come together in person, the time for active learning, skills practice, and deep reflection is maximized. Critically, adequate time should be allotted for faculty development activities that allow for debriefing, reflection, planning, and follow-up (Hall & Zierler, 2015). Utilizing time in this way is most meaningful to faculty and facilitates the transfer of the new knowledge and skills into interprofessional teaching and learning practice (Simmons et al., 2011).

FACULTY RECOGNITION FOR IMPLEMENTING AND FACILITATING INTERPROFESSIONAL EDUCATION

An important component to faculty development is recognizing the time and effort that faculty expend to implement and facilitate IPE, particularly since these efforts are typically undertaken in addition to regular faculty duties. Identifying nonmonetary strategies that acknowledge and document the contributions of faculty participation in implementing and evaluating IPE activities can be placed in a faculty member's academic file and used for career progression. Examples include personalized thank-you notes, letters to department chairs and supervisors, certificates of completion, and peer evaluations from colleagues and students. Assisting junior faculty in producing scholarship as a result of their faculty development training is another nonmonetary method of recognizing their efforts.

IMPLICATIONS FOR NURSING EDUCATION

Faculty development and institutionalization of IPE has implications for nursing education at the systems and individual levels. The IPEC Core Competency domains are designed for all health professions, and it is widely recognized that they should be taught interprofessionally. However, given the current siloing of health professions education, IPE requires more coordination of curricula across health professions schools and strategic partnerships between academia and practice. As the need for faculty development in IPE increases, IPE-competent faculty will likely be more invested to engage in efforts to coordinate health professions curricula.

As noted previously, the conceptual framework proposed by the IOM Consensus Committee report on the impact of IPE on collaborative practice and patient outcomes (IOM, 2015) highlights where the majority of IPE currently occurs (in the classroom) but suggests that the greatest opportunities to learn about CP is in the practice environment. Because the ultimate goal of IPE is to foster CP to improve the quality and safety of care, perhaps the greatest opportunity to learn this is in the clinical or community setting. Thus, single-profession schools that start with purposeful IPE in the practice environment with students from other programs within the same city or with practitioners may achieve competency in CP in a more meaningful way. To date, we do not know the dose, timing, or duration of IPE necessary to produce "collaborative practice-ready" nurses, and there are no data to suggest that IPE in the classroom improves CP or patient outcomes or that any skills are transferred to practice. Using the expanded Kirkpatrick model, described in detail in Chapter 2 (Reeves et al., 2015), IPE in the classroom is at the lower two levels of learning and is focused on changing knowledge, attitudes, and skills about interprofessional teamwork (IOM, 2015). Furthermore, the IOM proposed model for IP learning suggests that *early* practice experiences are the greatest opportunity to learn and support CP (IOM, 2015). This means that the majority of interprofessional learning may occur in clinical and practice settings, which in turn may necessitate more diversity and flexibility in how nursing education is delivered. Partnerships with the community and patients/families will also become more common to ensure that practice- or community-based joint learning opportunities occur. To achieve this, sites (and preceptors) will need to be developed in tandem with faculty development to support CP in visible and explicit ways.

Teaching the IPEC Core Competencies interprofessionally, particularly when schools are not located in academic health centers, requires creativity. Schools (and faculty) are looking to other non–health-related professions within their schools or are reaching out to other schools to cocreate activities that will provide their students with interprofessional learning opportunities. For example, nursing programs may partner with non–health-related disciplines, such as engineering, law, education, architecture, or public policy, to create opportunities that allow the *process* of IPE to occur so that students gain exposure to learning with and from others with different professional identities. The knowledge and skills gained from IPE faculty development programs will facilitate these creative opportunities.

At the individual level, teaching interprofessionally requires that faculty model interprofessional behavior by partnering with colleagues from other disciplines. To do that, faculty need opportunities to interact and collaborate with other faculty—and nursing schools may need to adapt current approaches to faculty development so that faculty can focus on developing and nurturing strategic partnerships. Teaching interprofessionally will also result in more interactive and student-driven learning in nursing.

EXAMPLES OF NATIONAL INTERPROFESSIONAL EDUCATION FACULTY DEVELOPMENT TRAINING PROGRAMS

A national train-the-trainer Interprofessional Faculty Development program was funded by the Josiah Macy Jr. Foundation in 2014. In collaboration with the National Center for Interprofessional Practice and Education (NCIPE), three training hubs will offer hands-on training (3.5 days in-person and follow-up coaching) for faculty who are already engaged and active with IPE at their institution. The three training hubs include the University of Washington, the University of Missouri (Columbia), and the University of Virginia at Arlington. The NCIPE will coordinate training for these three sites and will track data on outcomes of training. A certificate of completion and continuing education credits will be offered to interprofessional teams.

The University of Kansas has created a faculty development program for preceptors in primary care. The Preceptor Training Toolkit is located at the NCIPE website: https://nexusipe.org/preceptors-nexus. This toolkit includes a wide array of tools that support and enrich interprofessional practice to enhance patient care, as well as professional development opportunities for clinical preceptors who facilitate interprofessional teams of learners.

The IPEC Institute offers 3-day trainings twice per year for health professions faculty and their IPE colleagues. The Institute provides both quality time and dedicated space for guided learning, team-based planning activities, and consultation with experts and peers to emerge with a programmatic action plan for IPE. Other faculty development trainings are offered regionally in association with IPE meetings.

CONCLUSION

This chapter identified different areas of training needed to produce a competent IPE educator: an understanding and modeling of the IPE competences, specific training needs for effective facilitation of IPE learners (coaching, negotiating, resolving conflict, addressing hierarchy, and stereotypes), pedagogical approaches to teaching IPE for disparate learners, and mentoring for IPE leadership. It also addressed additional issues of relevance to faculty development: the need for support to create interprofessional curricula, areas to consider in implementing faculty development programs, and the importance of acknowledgment and rewards for participating in IPE being critical to remaining engaged. Competencies needed to be a skilled IPE educator are similar to those we are striving to develop in our students—and like students, faculty need the opportunity to develop and practice these skills. By working together collaboratively, faculty are modeling the behaviors needed in future healthcare professionals to ensure high-quality, cost-effective, and safe care.

References

Anderson E. S., Cox, D., & Thorpe, L. N. (2009). Preparation of educators involved in interprofessional education. *Journal of Interprofessional Care, 23*(1), 81–94.

Bjorke, G., & Haave, N. (2006). Crossing boundaries: Implementing interprofessional education into uniprofessional bachelor programmes. *Journal of Interprofessional Care, 20*, 641–653.

Bridges, D. R., Davidson, R. A. Odegard, P. S. Maki, I. V., & Tomkowiak, J. (2011). Interprofessional collaboration: Three best practice models of interprofessional education. *Medical Education Online, 16*. Published online April 8, 2011. doi:10.3402/ meo.v16i0.6035

Buring, S. M., Bhushan, A., Brazeau, G., Conway, S., Hansen, L., & Westberg, S. (2009). Keys to successful implementation of interprofessional education: Learning location, faculty development, and curricular themes. *American Journal of Pharmaceutical Education, 73*(4), 1–11.

Craddock, D., O'Halloran, C., McPherson, K., Hean, S., & Hammick, M. (2013). A top-down approach impedes the use of theory? Interprofessional educational leaders' approaches to curriculum development and the use of learning theory. *Journal of Interprofessional Care, 27*(1), 65–72.

Dematteo, D., & Reeves, S. (2011). A critical examination of the role of appreciative inquiry within an interprofessional education initiative. *Journal of Interprofessional Care, 25*(3), 203–208.

Freeman, S., Wright, A., & Lindqvist, S. (2010). Facilitator training for educators involved in interprofessional learning. *Journal of Interprofessional Care, 24*(4), 375–385.

Freeth D, Hammick, M, Reeves, S., Koppel, I., & Barr, H. (2005). Effective interprofessional education. *Development, delivery and evaluation.* Oxford, England: Blackwell.

Hall, L. W., & Zierler, B. K. (2015). Interprofessional Education and Practice Guide No. 1: Developing faculty to effectively facilitate interprofessional education. *Journal of Interprofessional Care, 29*(1), 3–7.

Hanna, E., Soren, B., Telner, D., MacNeill, H., Lowe, M., & Reeves, S. (2013). Flying blind: The experience of online interprofessional facilitation. *Journal of Interprofessional Care, 27*(4), 298–304.

Howkins, E., & Bray, J. (2008). *Preparing for interprofessional teaching: Theory and practice.* Boca Raton, FL: CRC Press.

Institute of Medicine. (2015). *Measuring the impact of interprofessional education (IPE) on collaborative practice and patient outcomes.* Washington DC: National Academies Press.

Interprofessional Education Collaborative Expert Panel. (2011). *Core competencies for interprofessional collaborative practice: Report of an expert panel.* Washington, DC: Interprofessional Education Collaborative.

Kreitner, R., & Kinicki, A. (2008). *Organizational behavior* (8th ed.). Boston: McGraw-Hill/Irwin.

Oandasan, I., & Reeves, S. (2005). Key elements for interprofessional education Part 1: The learner, the educator and the learning context. *Journal of Interprofessional Care, 19*, 21–38.

Owen, J., & Schmitt, M. (2013). Integrating interprofessional education into continuing education: A planning process for continuing interprofessional education programs. *Journal of Continuing Education in the Health Professions, 33*(2), 109–117.

Reeves, S., Boet, S., Zierler, B., Kitto, S. (2015). Interprofessional education and practice guide no. 3: Evaluating interprofessional education. *Journal of Interprofessional Care, 29*(4), 305–312.

Reeves, S., & Freeth, D. (2002). The London training ward: An innovative interprofessional learning initiative. *Journal of Interprofessional Care, 16*(1), 41–52.

Reeves, S., Lewin, S., Espin, S., & Zwarenstein, M. (2010). *Interprofessional teamwork for health and social care.* Oxford, England: Wiley-Blackwell.

Ruiz, M., Ezer, H., & Purden, M. (2013). Exploring the nature of facilitating interprofessional learning: Findings from an exploratory study. *Journal of Interprofessional Care, 27*(6), 489–495.

Sargeant, J. (2009). Theories to aid understanding and implementation of interprofessional education. *Journal of Continuing Education in the Health Professions, 29*(3), 178–184.

Shrader, S., Mauldin, M., Hammad, S., Mitcham, M., & Blue, A. (2015). Developing a comprehensive faculty development program to promote interprofessional education, practice and research at a free-standing academic health science center. *Journal of Interprofessional Care, 29*(2), 165–167.

Simmons, B., Oandasan, I., Soklaradis, S., Esdaile, M, Barker, K., Kwan, D., et al. (2011). Evaluating the effectiveness of an interprofessional education faculty development course: The transfer of interprofessional learning to the academic and clinical practice setting. *Journal of Interprofessional Care, 25*, 156–157.

Speakman, E., Tagliareni, E., Sherburne, A., & Sicks, S. (2016). *Guide to effective interprofessional education experiences in nursing.* Available at http://www.nln.org

Steinert, Y. (2005). Learning together to teach together: Interprofessional education and faculty development. *Journal of Interprofessional Care, 19*(Suppl. 1), 60–75.

Steinert, Y. (2012). Perspectives on faculty development: Aiming for 6/6 by 2020. *Perspectives in Medical Education, 1*(1), 31–42.

Steinert, Y., MacDonald, M. E., Boillat, M., Elizov, M., Meterissian, S., Razack, S., et al. (2010). Faculty development: If you build it, they will come. *Medical Education, 44*(9), 900–907.

Steinert, Y., Mann, K., Centeno, A., Dolmans, D., Spencer, J., Gelula, M., et al. (2006). A systematic review of faculty development initiatives designed to improve teaching effectiveness in medical education: BEME Guide No 8. *Medical Teacher, 28*(6), 497–526.

Thistlethwaite, J., Moran, M., & World Health Organization Study Group on Interprofessional Education and Collaborative Practice. (2010). Learning outcomes for interprofessional education (IPE): Literature review and synthesis. *Journal of Interprofessional Care, 24*(5), 503–513.

Wenger, E. (1998). *Communities of practice: Learning, meaning, and identity.* Cambridge, UK: Cambridge University Press.

Willgerodt, M. A., Blakeney, E. A., Brock, D. M., Liner, D., Murphy, N., & Zierler, B. (2015). Interprofessional Education and Practice Guide No. 4: Developing and sustaining interprofessional education at an academic health center. *Journal of Interprofessional Care,* Advance online publication. doi:10.3109/13561820.2015.1039117

4

The Benefits of the Patient Educator/ Mentor to Maximize Student Learning in Interprofessional Teams

Lauren Collins, MD

Tracey Vause Earland, PhD (c), MS, OTR/L

Sarah Dallas, BA

Chelsea Gorman Lytle, BSN, RN

As described in previous chapters, there is a general consensus among health providers, policymakers, health organizations, and consumers that interprofessional team approaches promote effective collaboration and patient-centered care throughout the healthcare system (Singla, MacKinnon, MacKinnon, Younis, & Field, 2004; Barr, Koppel, Reeves, Hammick, & Freeth, 2005). Interprofessional education (IPE) is widely advocated as a key element to promote an effective, redesigned healthcare system. Health providers are beginning to recognize that no single profession has the means to address today's complex patient issues exclusively. The Institute of Medicine (IOM) has stated that "all health professionals should be educated to deliver patient-centered care as members of an interdisciplinary team, emphasizing evidence-based practice, quality improvement approaches, and informatics" (Institute of Medicine [IOM], 2003, p. 3). Subsequently, the World Health Organization (WHO) has been eager to advance the international IPE agenda (Oandasan & Reeves, 2005), supporting the IOM notion that well-trained interprofessional teams can make substantial improvements in quality of care and an IPE model will produce health professionals with the necessary attitudes, skills, and knowledge to work collaboratively with team members, the patient/client, and family. To reach this standard of practice, the IOM and WHO advocate for structured, well-designed interprofessional curriculum in health professions education.

Educators and national nursing organizations such as the National League for Nursing (NLN), the American Association of Colleges of Nursing (AACN), the American Nurses Association (ANA), and the American Organization of Nurse Executives (AONE), as well as other health professions organizations such as the Association of American Medical Colleges (AAMC), the American Association of Colleges of Pharmacy (AACP), and the American Physical Therapy Association (APTA), are increasingly exhorting IPE. Most health professions education now includes IPE in accreditation standards, and academic programs must adhere to the requirements published by the institution's respective accrediting body by incorporating IPE within the curriculum. In 2012, a comparative analysis on IPE accreditation standards among various health professions institutes in the United States was conducted. The Commission on Collegiate Nursing Education and the Accreditation Council for Pharmacy Education documents contained 77 percent (46/60) of accountable IPE statements that mandate achieving a specific IPE learner outcome (Zorek & Raehl, 2012). The authors concluded that based on the frequency of accreditation standards reflecting IPE competencies, nursing and pharmacy graduates may be the most prepared for interprofessional collaborative practice (CP).

As noted in Chapter 3, classroom-based activities are wonderful instructional approaches to teaching the tenets of IPE and helping students to achieve the four IPEC Core Competencies. But part of an essential component to IPE and teamwork is placing the patient at the center of collaborative care. Conceptually, patients are active members of the interprofessional healthcare team, sharing their values, preferences, and goals. In fact, patients are the decisive justification for the origin of interprofessional CP. Collaborative patient-centered practice is the model for which everyone on the team—including the patient—exchange information, share decision making, problem solve, and work together. The biopsychosocial model of care acknowledges the patient as the expert on his or her personal and cultural background and values the patient's perspective of the illness experience. For nursing, there is an opportunity for the profession to meet the demands for patient-centered care services (Terrien & Hale, 2014). Nurses have key roles as team members and facilitators of integrated, patient-centered interventions. If patient-centered care is truly a hallmark of interprofessional collaborative care, then educational programs should actively incorporate patient educators into their professional education.

PATIENT INVOLVEMENT IN EDUCATIONAL CURRICULUM

Patient educators/mentors/instructors have contributed to health education for close to 50 years (Terrien & Hale, 2014). Patient instructors were seen as "expert in their condition; exemplars of their medical condition, and facilitators of professional skills and attitudes" (Costello & Horne, 2001, p. 95). The use of patients as healthcare educators and partners is increasingly recognized as a successful method for delivering patient-centered education (Towle & Godolphin, 2013; IOM, 2014; Fulmer & Gaines, 2014). The earlier that students can hear the "lived experiences" of their patient educator and understand the patient's perspective, the better they can integrate the patient's narrative into their practice (Terrien & Hale, 2014). This experience gives students an opportunity to engage in meaningful interactions and increase their awareness of the patient's reality. Students hear firsthand the challenges of negotiating the health system; the impact of their condition on life goals, family, and career paths; and other insights on their quality of life (Giordano et al., 2013). Partnering students with patients early and consistently throughout their training has garnered increasing attention as an ideal format for a redesigned health professions educational system.

Over the years, there has been a wide range of patient involvement in educating future practitioners. Towle et al. (2010) did a literature review on active patient involvement in health professions education. The researchers noted the difficulty in searching the literature due to the lack of standardized terminology describing the role of the patient. However, Towle et al. (2010) found a spectrum of patient involvement, including the following: (a) the patient serving as a volunteer in a clinical setting; (b) the patient sharing his or her experience with students, within a faculty-directed curriculum; (c) patient-teachers being involved in teaching or evaluating students; (d) patient-teachers being equal partners in student education, evaluation, and curriculum development; and (e) the patient being involved at the institutional level in addition to sustained involvement as a patient-teacher in education (Towle et al., 2010). These are just a few key roles that community volunteers with various conditions and/or disabilities have served in nursing, medical, and health professions education.

BENEFITS OF THE PATIENT EDUCATOR/MENTOR

Interactions with patient educators/mentors can be a valuable learning experience for nursing and other students in the health professions as they are exposed to the patient's perspectives, goals and values, and what they deem important. These encounters offer the student the opportunity to partner with the patient educator and develop skills supporting collaborative, patient-centered care. Studies indicate that students who partner with patients demonstrate greater understanding of the lived experiences of patients and use less interpersonal distancing (Wood & Wilson-Barnett, 1999). Using a patient educator model, students learn to facilitate and embrace patient choice regarding care and develop advocacy skills for their patient (Norman et al., 1996). There is also evidence that patient educator/mentor partnerships have lasting impact on students' interpersonal skills, empathic understanding, and ability to individualize care based on the patient's perceived needs (Wood & Wilson-Barnett, 1999; Klein, Tracy, Kitchener, & Walker, 1999).

The role of patient educator/mentor is a mutual benefit to the patient as well. Many patient educators choose to volunteer their time out of a genuine interest in training future health professionals. Patient educators want to give back to the community by sharing their experiential knowledge of illness to future practitioners. Patient mentors have expressed enjoyment in the companionship of students. This partnership fosters raised self-esteem, empowerment, and opportunities to understand and gain new insights on their life challenges (Towle et al., 2010).

Partnership with the patient educator/mentor enables the student to learn directly from the patient and is at the core of CP. Coordinated educational curricula involving patient educators and students in interprofessional health have the potential to promote meaningful partnerships and achieve the goal of patient-centered care.

A CASE STUDY IN PARTNERING WITH PATIENTS: THE JEFFERSON HEALTH MENTORS PROGRAM

To address the gap in team-based chronic illness care education, an interprofessional team of faculty at our university developed a longitudinal IPE curriculum called the *Jefferson Health Mentors Program* (JHMP). This program is required for all first- and second-year students from the colleges of nursing, medicine, pharmacy, physician assistant, occupational therapy, physical therapy, and couple and family therapy. Interprofessional student teams are paired with a "health mentor," a community volunteer living with one or more chronic health conditions or impairments who is interested in sharing his or her personal narrative with a team of students in the health professions. The health mentor is identified as an "educator" as well as a team member (Collins et al., 2011).

The 2-year JHMP curriculum consists of four key modules, plus orientation sessions at the beginning of each year and interprofessional small group sessions following each module. These modules include the following: (a) Obtaining a Comprehensive Life and Health History, (b) Preparing a Self-Management Support Plan for Wellness and Healthy Behavior, (c) Assessing Patient Safety, and (d) Interprofessional Education and Practice. Initially conceived by a representative team of faculty and student champions in 2006, the JHMP gained approval from the curriculum committees of each profession at Jefferson and was first implemented in 2007. Despite undergoing multiple rounds of continuous quality improvement and curricular revisions, three overarching goals have guided this longitudinal mentorship program since inception: (a) students will understand the perspective of the patient and value patient-centered care, (b) students will understand and value the roles and contributions of various members of the interprofessional healthcare team, and (c) students will appreciate how a person's health conditions and impairments interact with personal and environmental factors (Collins et al., 2013).

JHMP as an Experiential Learning Opportunity: Chelsea's Personal Perspective

The JHMP focuses on expanding student understanding of the unique roles and responsibilities of each health professional within a healthcare team by utilizing a variety of experiential, team-based learning exercises. In fact, the use of experiential learning opportunities helps the nursing student prepare for the demands of a dynamic workforce (Della Ratta, 2015). Although it is clear that experiential learning opportunities can have a profound effect on the student's professional acumen, using reflection activities can provide a rich understanding of the impact of these experiences on the student's personal transformation. The following is coauthor Chelsea Gorham Lytle's perspective:

> During my time at Jefferson College of Nursing at Thomas Jefferson University, Interprofessional Education (IPE) has become a passion of mine. I believe that all health professions students should be exposed to collaborative practice as early and as often as possible. At Jefferson, we enter the Health Mentors Program (HMP), a longitudinal IPE curriculum, almost as soon as we matriculate into our field of study. As first-year students, we are placed in small, interprofessional teams and each team is paired with a health mentor who is living with at least one chronic illness or impairment. We completed four modules over the two-year period and met in small groups before and after each module.
>
> Our first meeting was held in the fall of my first semester at Jefferson. Several teams met together in small groups led by a faculty facilitator. The first part of this meeting was spent getting to know the members of my team. There were five of us: two medical students, one occupational therapy student, one couple and family therapy student, and me, a nursing student. At first, it was clear that we had very little idea what students in the other professions knew and what their roles would be within our team. Under the guidance of the facilitator, we discussed the upcoming first module of the HMP.
>
> Module One consisted of meeting with our mentor for the first time, conducting an interview, and recording a complete health history. Before our mentor arrived, my team met to

discuss how we would conduct the interview. We divided the health history form we had been given into sections that seemed most relevant to each of our roles and decided to take a conversational approach to the interview. When our Mentor arrived, it quickly became obvious that we would have no difficulties getting her to share her story with us. CW was a 56-year-old African-American female living with type two diabetes. She explained that teaching was her passion. She was active in diabetes education groups, attended conferences, was active in her church, and volunteered at a local school. She was very knowledgeable about her condition and how to control it through diet and medication. She had no issues with mobility and stated that she was eager to "get up and go" every day. CW shared that she was divorced and lived with her special needs daughter who was also diabetic. She had two other children with whom she had little contact. When we asked her what kind of support system she had, CW told us that God and the church were her strength and that she did not need any other support.

Throughout that first interview, our team worked together cohesively. After CW left, we had a chance to discuss the meeting. Our entire group was relieved that we had been matched with such a loquacious and enthusiastic mentor. We quickly realized that each of us had taken different meaning from many of the statements that CW had made. This helped us to discuss our roles in more depth than had previously been possible. Later that semester, we met again in a group of a few other teams to discuss our experiences with Module One. We discovered that not all mentors had been as forthcoming as ours and not all teams had worked as cohesively. The group spent some time discussing possible reasons behind any issues that had arisen and brainstorming ways to address them.

The next semester, we met again to prepare for Module Two. We learned about different elements of wellness and working with our Mentors to create wellness goals. A few weeks later, my team met with CW for the second time. We began by discussing in general what had been going on in her life. She shared that although her physical health had remained the same, she had begun to experience severe anxiety. She had been to see a psychologist twice, but was not planning to return. At this point, the couple and family therapy student took charge. He strongly encouraged CW to continue seeing her therapist and began to ask questions about the cause of her anxiety. It became clear that there were two major causes for her distress: her estrangement from her children and feeling unsafe in her home. The occupational therapy student and I questioned her further about the safety of her home environment. CW told us that while she felt safe while she was in her home, her neighborhood frightened her. We worked with her to develop goals that would help her feel safer at home and work toward improving her communication and trust. We also helped her identify strengths that were already promoting wellness in her life. Before CW left that day, she had also agreed to continue seeing her psychologist. Our final group meeting of Year One consisted of discussing the goals we had developed with our Mentors, sharing how our team had worked and grown together, and examining how our Mentors' conditions had changed over the course of a year.

At the beginning of our second year, we met again to prepare for Module Three. We reconnected as a team and discussed what was happening in each of our programs. During this session, we learned about home visits and medication reviews and prepared to meet with our Mentors for the last time. Unfortunately, CW was unable to have us visit her home, but she agreed to bring pictures to help us discuss potential safety issues. When CW arrived for our final meeting, it was obvious that her physical condition had changed. She was no longer able to easily climb stairs or walk long distances. She told us that the cortisone injections she had been receiving were no longer relieving the pain in her knee. This new information changed the focus of our safety review. From the pictures, we learned that CW had to climb uneven steps with only one hand rail to enter her home. She did not have a shower chair or a grab bar in her bathroom and told us that she had been sitting on the edge of the tub to shower. We let CW know that she should speak to her primary care provider about getting a referral to an occupational therapist who could help her find the right shower chair. We also helped her contact her landlord who agreed to help install a shower chair, grab bar, and an extra handrail. Before CW left that day, she told us that she wished that we could be her real health care team.

At the beginning of my last semester at Jefferson, we had another small group meeting to discuss the new Module Four. The HMP had responded to students' desire for a more clinically relevant approach to IPE by redesigning this module to give students the chance to participate in a variety of learning activities that explored how collaborative practice works in real-world settings. During my time at Jefferson, I had been involved in the creation and implementation of IPE Grand Rounds, which was one of the learning activities incorporated into this module. This program increases interaction between real-world collaborative practice teams and health professions students in the form of a panel discussion. I decided to use our Palliative Care Team event as my Module Four learning activity. The team consisted of a social worker, a member of the pastoral care team, two physicians, and a nurse practitioner. The team began by explaining what palliative care was and their team's role in the hospital. They then shared a case study, encouraging audience participation throughout the presentation. The team closed by answering questions from the audience. I was impressed by the team's honesty, communication skills, and obvious respect for the roles that each member of their team played. Despite their success as a collaborative practice team, they shared the challenges that they had faced and encouraged all of the students present to "do it better" than they had been able to.

After attending this learning activity, I completed an individual reflection essay. Although it primarily focused on the learning activity I had attended, it also provided a chance to reflect on my experience with HMP as a whole. I can honestly say that the time that I have spent in pursuit of interprofessional education has been one of the most rewarding and clinically relevant parts of my nursing education.

Assessment of the JHMP

Trying to keep pace with ongoing changes in practice redesign, the JHMP is a dynamic IPE program that undergoes an iterative process of quality improvement each year, searching for new and better ways to reform health professions education and promote an integrated approach to patient-centered care. Outcome evaluation includes both quantitative and qualitative methods. Quantitative evaluation tools are used to gather data at baseline and at the end of the 2-year program. Data analysis leads to both identification of program successes and needs for future improvements. Course evaluation data has been increasingly positive over the past 8 years with each round of quality improvement. With the implementation of the updated and revised curriculum this academic year, the JHMP has again received very high student course evaluations; the majority of students from all seven professions agreed that the IPE modules helped in their achievement of program goals (Roy et al., 2016). Ratings for nursing students were 96 percent agreement at the end of Year One and 97 percent at the end of Year Two.

Sample Nursing Student Feedback

In addition to quantitative data from course evaluations and surveys, open-ended responses have provided a unique insight into the nursing student experience in the JHMP. Sample quotes are included in Boxes 4.1 and 4.2. In addition to voluntarily completing the module evaluation, Year Two students were required to submit a

BOX 4.1

Nursing Student Feedback on JHMP Module 2 (Preparing a Self-Management Support Plan for Wellness and Healthy Behavior)

Did the visit with your health mentor for Module 2 contribute to your achievement of program goals and objectives?
(Student teams met with health mentor, discussed dimensions of wellness, and developed SMART goals.)

"It was interesting to be able to gather information from our health mentor and then Figure out what was important to her and what she wanted to work on. We factored in personal and environmental factors as well as barriers to develop a SMART goal."

Open-ended evaluation question asking students to list one thing that they liked or learned from their experience in Module 2:
"I really enjoyed that everyone brings a different point of view to the table. As the health mentor is talking everyone's mind is working differently and thinking of interventions and strategies that they learned about in class or in their clinical experiences. Having a plan made up by people from 5 different medical disciplines is a lot stronger than a plan made up from just one type of medical standpoint."

"I liked hearing about all of the other teams' approaches to wellbeing and how they molded each wellness goal to fit the individualized needs of their mentors. It opened my mind up to more interventions and ways I can help out my patients in the future that I would not have thought of if I hadn't listened to other team members speak about their experiences."

"I liked hearing each member's input, while we were completing the assignment. As a nursing student, I valued educating the patient and telling her signs to look for if she was pushing herself too hard during her workout, whereas the OT student focused more on safety, and the med students were more concerned about the patient's ability to complete her SMART goal giv[en] her whole history. Everyone offered something unique and it is cool to see what each profession values."

BOX 4.2

Nursing Student Feedback on JHMP Module 4 (Interprofessional Education and Practice)

Did the Interprofessional Education and Practice (IPEP) Learning Activity for Module 4 that you selected contribute to your achievement of program goals and objectives?
"[The] SAHP [Shadowing an Alternative Healthcare Professional] activity helped me to see more clearly how each member of [the] healthcare team [is] trying to achieve same goal."

"The presentation [IPE Grand Rounds featuring a panel presentation from the Senior Adult Oncology Team] allowed me to [g]et a different view of the field of oncology and the team's approach towards the coordination of care."

Open-ended evaluation question asking students to list one thing that they liked or learned from their experience in Module 4:
"Learned how the interaction between professionals from different disciplines can greatly impact the development of individualized plan of care for patient."

"I liked how IPE Grand Rounds showed real life interprofessional teamwork in the hospital setting."

"Teamwork and respect for team member's area of expertise, and maintaining open communication with other team members."

reflection essay describing the Interprofessional Education and Practice activity in which they participated and reflecting on their experience in the program and with their health mentor. Additional qualitative analysis of student reflection essays has demonstrated an even more marked effect of the program on students' appreciation of the challenges and benefits of team-based person-centered care (Giordano et al., 2013; Roy et al., 2016). One observed benefit of this program is the shift in student values regarding the provision of healthcare. In the written reflections, faculty have noted a culture change from wanting to "fix" a patient's chronic condition to attempting to better understand the context of the person's life experiences before and after diagnosis of one or more chronic conditions. Students describe adopting a new perspective of caring for patients with chronic conditions. For example, one student wrote:

> When going to my mentor's house, I realized how his disability completely changed every aspect of his life. He had to make many modifications to his home and continues to find new modifications that he can make to increase the ease with which he lives on a daily basis. Things that we constantly take for granted and take 5 minutes to perform, take him 20 plus minutes and he often needs to use adaptive equipment to complete ADLs.

One nursing student who participated in a Schwartz Round on the topic of "Aftershock: Feeling Distressed When Your Case Takes an Unexpected Turn" said:

> I learned so much from attending this panel. I realize that although I may be tired and anxious to leave at the end of a long and difficult shift, especially if a case took a bad turn, it is highly important to meet up with my team members. I will do this moving forward in my professional practice, not just because I understand that tragedy is too much to cope with alone. I want to feel supported, and I want my team to feel supported by me. I do not want to lose sight of the fact that my career involves human lives, and sometimes those lives are cut short for whatever reason.

Providing the opportunity for students to participate in classroom learning–based collaborative settings helped students see the full picture and realize the goals of the JHMP. In one reflection essay, a nursing student stated the following:

> I am directly affected by my participation in the health mentors program because it helps me find my voice in the crowd of other health professions.... Now I will feel confident when conversing with doctors and other members of the healthcare team by taking what I learned from my health mentors experience and applying it to real-life situations.

In another essay, a nursing student reflected on the importance of clear communication and being on the same page as your team members:

> This is helpful when applying it to healthcare because so many professions listen to the same "story" (the patient's medical history) and each of us can choose to focus on a different underlying theme of [the patient's] history. This is why it is super helpful and important for all health professions to collaborate together with the development of the patient plan of care and implementing that plan. It is crucial that everyone's patient information overlaps so that every member is on the same page when caring for a patient.

Another major benefit of the JHMP is the collaboration that has naturally developed within interprofessional student teams. By bringing students from the various programs together to complete JHMP visits and assignments, they establish relationships with peers and across professions that rarely occurred in previous years. One student wrote:

> From the moment we met we had a mutual understanding that although in different disciplines with different demands we would all work together at these assignments. We also were very open to learning about one another's discipline, our program's demands, and what we were learning in order to better understand one another and how we think.

Written reflections reveal emergent awareness of and respect for the scope, rigor, and demands of their fellow team members' training, practice, and expertise. A 2013 study on student attitudes toward healthcare teams demonstrated a significant improvement in attitudes comparing baseline to the end of the 2-year JHMP scores (Giordano et al., 2013). A noticeable shift in campus culture has resulted in students now expecting to work with peers from other professional programs, where 8 years ago most students might never even have met colleagues from other training programs on campus. Graduating students who have completed the JHMP are including this experience in their resumes and personal statements as a highlight of their education.

Sample Health Mentor Feedback

Recently the health mentors were surveyed using a mixed methods study and reported an overall high satisfaction with the JHMP along with a reported increased motivation to make and maintain healthy behaviors. High satisfaction levels from working with interprofessional student teams were reported; substantial improvement in the management of their health conditions and improvements in overall health status was relayed. Examples of positive responses from surveyed health mentors include statements such as these: *"I am more conscious of healthy choices, food, etc.," "I've been more active on a regular basis," "I am willing to listen and take charge of my health,"* and *"I feel more accountability to follow through with my health goals."* Self-reported knowledge gained by health mentors from student teams included issues related to strategies to improve home safety, self-care, medication usage and safety, nutrition, exercise, sleep patterns, and goal setting. Further studies are now underway to determine if the patient-reported outcomes of our health mentors correlate with objective health measures (Umland, Collins, Lin, Baronner, & Giordano, in review).

Implementation Strategies for Health Mentor Programming: Challenges and Lessons Learned

Particular challenges with implementing a broad IPE curriculum like the JHMP include programmatic and scheduling logistics, student perceptions, and at times the health and busy schedules of the health mentors themselves. During the cycles of continuous quality improvement of this curriculum, it has been critical for JHMP modules to not contribute to curriculum overload or repetitiveness in any particular profession's curricula. Module content was designed to meet curricular objectives for all participating professions and was integrated into the existing profession-specific courses. Logistics of coordinating each profession's academic and examination schedules with scheduling dates for orientation, mentor visits, assignment due dates, and interprofessional team debriefing sessions are an ongoing challenge. An interprofessional faculty, student, and Health Mentor Steering Committee now begins the scheduling process 6 to 12 months before the start of the academic year. In addition, the use of "university time," a 2-hour time block during which no classes are scheduled, for hosting health mentor visits and for interprofessional small group (IPE) sessions emphasizes to students and faculty the value placed on JHMP by our university.

Another primary challenge for this IPE curricular innovation was the initial lack of a common language across health professions regarding health and wellness. This challenge was addressed in 2010 by incorporating the International Classification of Functioning, Disability and Health framework (ICF) throughout the 2-year JHMP curriculum (World Health Organization [WHO], 2001). Students and mentors now use the ICF framework to communicate more effectively as a team and to better understand the interaction of a person with his or her health conditions, social roles, and environment.

Ultimately, the success of the JHMP has rested on the combined efforts of the 250 volunteer health mentors, the assistance from more than 10 community organizations (including public health agencies, local senior centers, senior housing facilities, and retirement communities that help to recruit volunteer health mentors), institutional support from Thomas Jefferson University, and the collaboration of seven professions (including 22 courses, more than 40 faculty, and approximately 1,300 students per year). A true measure of success, the JHMP has now been successfully adapted and implemented at many other institutions over the past 5 years.

ENGAGING NURSING STUDENTS IN INTERPROFESSIONAL EDUCATION

A critical lesson learned in introducing and sustaining the JHMP is the value of engaging student leaders from each profession. Each year, JHMP faculty invite two students from each profession to serve as course liaisons. Course liaisons serve many roles, including providing curricular feedback; improving communication among faculty, health mentors, and student peers; and serving as interprofessional leaders and advocates. To date, student course liaisons have played a key role in re-engineering the JHMP by encouraging increased use of technology, such as adoption of Team Wiki sites for posting of module instructions and completing team assignments, along with gaining support for an optional online small group discussion. Student course liaisons have also successfully advocated for increased exposure to roles of various health professionals and have driven curricular changes in the JHMP toward increasing student exposure to real-world CP teams early on in their training programs. Graduating students who have completed the JHMP are including this experience in their resumes and personal statements as a highlight of their education. Alumni of this longitudinal IPE program have informed us that they have a "leg up" in the job market because of their experience in team-based collaborative care.

In addition to serving as JHMP course liaisons, nursing and other students in the health professions have become increasingly engaged in institution-wide IPE and CP initiatives, including curricular, cocurricular, and extracurricular activities. Students have led the production and editing of a health mentor newsletter that is published each semester and designed to provide health mentors with information about upcoming

JHMP events and additionally has health education columns. Students now also participate as editors on the Jefferson Center for Interprofessional Education Newsletter Editorial Board and serve as steering committee members for Thomas Jefferson University's interprofessional Schwartz Rounds. Over the past few years, students have taken an active role in the development of an extracurricular program called *JeffCHAT*, a student-run interprofessional program designed to promote reflection and foster compassion among future healthcare providers, which is modeled after Schwartz Rounds but dedicated only to student participants. In addition, in the past academic year, a new student-led organziation called the *Jefferson Students for Interprofessional Education* was formed and led by an elected student president from the college of nursing. This new organization is advancing IPE initiatives across our institution, adding monthly interactive IPE Grand Rounds that feature CP teams and promoting IPE research. During this past year, students have participated in a recent institution-wide IPE retreat, helping to craft a new mission statement for our IPE center and providing invaluable feedback to guide our institution's commitment to advanced training in IPE and CP.

Student leadership and engagement has been increasingly recognized locally and nationally. Recently, a team of our interprofessional students were selected to participate in a nationally funded Hot Spotting Learning Collaborative, which involves teaching teams of future health practitioners the challenges faced by complex patients interfacing with the current healthcare system. These students from different health professions work together to learn how to identify "superutilizers" and deepen their understanding of the factors that lead to high healthcare utilization and multiple readmissions. This past academic year, four students, including one from the college of nursing, were recognized with awards for excellence in IPE. In addition, student leaders in IPE have been involved in numerous research projects on campus and have participated in the presentation and publication of more than 20 peer-reviewed abstracts and manuscripts. By allowing students to have ownership of their own learning in IPE and to feel that their input is valued by our institution, many of our students have emerged as leaders in the field of IPE.

CONCLUSION

The JHMP described in this chapter serves as a case study for how to maximize IPE through experiential learning using patients as educators. Although the JHMP is unique in scale (with more than 1,300 students participating each academic year and more than 4,100 graduates of the program), it has been replicated successfully at numerous other institutions and can be implemented on a smaller scale. The JHMP success can largely be attributed to the support of our volunteer health mentors, faculty, and student leaders. Key to success has been the willingness of faculty, students, and health mentors to learn together, as well as learn from each other. Communication, mutual respect, flexibility, and an unwavering commitment to the ideal of interprofessional person-centered education have become hallmarks of the JHMP. Implementation of this large IPE program requires coordination; continuous quality improvement; and institutional, faculty, and student buy-in. Since process and outcome evaluations are incorporated as key elements of the overall JHMP assessment plan, the JHMP team has been able to ensure continuous quality improvement over the past 8 years. By incorporating a program like the JHMP, other institutions will be primed to meet expanding IPE accreditation standards, and their nursing students will graduate equipped to serve as effective members of the patient-centered healthcare team. Teamwork and interpersonal competencies are essential skills for nurses and a prerequiste to high-quality patient care (Della Ratta, 2015).

References

Barr, H., Koppel, I., Reeves, S., Hammick, M., & Freeth, D. (2005). Effective interprofessional education: Argument, assumption and evidence. Oxford, England: Blackwell.

Collins, L., Ankam, N., Antony, R., Hewston, L., Koeuth, S., Smith, K., et al. (2013). Preparing students for collaborative practice: An overview of the 2012 Jefferson Health Mentors Program. *MedEdPORTAL*. Retrieved June 6, 2016, from https://www.meded portal.org/publication/9312

Collins, L. G., Arenson, C. A., Jerpbak, C., Dressel, R., Kane, P., Antony, R., et al. (2011). Transforming chronic care education: A longitudinal interprofessional mentorship curriculum. *Journal of Interprofessional Care, 25*(3), 228–230.

Costello, J., & Horne, M. (2001). Patient as teachers? An evaluative study of patients' involvement in classroom teaching. *Nurse Education in Practice, 1*, 94–102.

Della Ratta, C. B. (2015). Flipping the classroom with team-based learning in undergraduate nursing education. *Nurse Educator, 40*(2), 71–74.

Fulmer, T., & Gaines, M. (2014). Partnering with patients, families, and communities to link interprofessional practice and education. Proceedings of a conference sponsored by the Josiah Macy Jr. Foundation, New York.

Giordano, C., Arenson, C., Lyons, K., Collins, L., Umland, E., Smith, K., et al. (2013). Effect of the Health Mentors Program on student attitudes toward team care. *Journal of Allied Health, 42*(2), 120–124.

Institute of Medicine. (2003). *Health professions education: A bridge to quality*. Washington, DC: The National Academics Press.

Institute of Medicine. (2014). *Partnering with patients to drive shared decisions, better value, and care improvement: Workshop Proceedings*. Washington, DC: National Academies Press.

Klein, S., Tracy, D., Kitchener, H. C., & Walker, L. G. (1999). The effects of the participation of patients with cancer in teaching communication skills to medical undergraduates: A randomized study with follow-up after 2 years. *European Journal of Cancer, 35*, 1448–1456.

Norman, I. J., Redfern, S., Bodley, D., Holroyd, S., Smith, C., & White, E. (1996). *The changing educational needs of mental health and learning disability nurses.* London: English National Board for Nursing, Midwifery and Health Visiting.

Roy, V., Collins, L. G., Sokas, C. M., Lim, E., Umland, E., Speakman, E., et al. (2016). Student reflections on interprofessional education: Moving from concepts to collaboration. *Journal of Allied Health, 45*(2), 109–112.

Singla, D. L., MacKinnon, G. E. III, MacKinnon, K. J., Younis, W., & Field, B. (2004). Interdisciplinary approach to teaching medication adherence to pharmacy and osteopathic medical students. *Journal of the American Osteopathic Association, 104*, 127–132.

Terrien, J., & Hale, J. (2014). Patients as educators: Contemporary application of an old educational strategy to promote patient-centered care. *Journal of Nursing Education and Practice, 4*, 104–113.

Towle, A., & Godolphin, W. (2013). Patients as educators: Interprofessional learning for patient-centered care. *Medical Teacher, 35*(3), 219–225.

Towle, A., Bainbridge, L., Godolphin, W., Katz, A., Kline, C., Lown, B., et al. (2010). Active patient involvement in the education of health professionals. *Medical Education, 44*(1), 64–74.

Umland, E., Collins, L., Lin, E., Baronner E., & Giordano C. (in review). Health mentor reported outcomes and perceptions of student team performance in a longitudinal interprofessional education (IPE) program. *Journal of Allied Health.*

Wood, J., & Wilson-Barnett, J. (1999). The influence of user involvement on the learning of mental health nursing students. *NT Research, 4,* 257–270.

World Health Organization. (2001). *International classification of functioning, disability and health (ICF).* Geneva, Switzerland: Author. Training materials available at http://www.who.int/classifications/icf/en/

Zorek, J., & Raehl, C. (2012). Interprofessional education accreditation standards in the USA: A comparative analysis. *Journal of Interprofessional Care.* E-pub September 6, 2012. doi:10.3109/13561820.2012.718295

5

Mobilization and Organizing Interprofessional Education and Collaborative Practice: Examining the Challenges and Opportunities

Mary T. Bouchaud, PhD, MSN, CNS, RN, CRRN

Shoshana Sicks, EDM, AB, EdD (S)

Catherine Mills

By nature, interprofessional education (IPE) cannot be done alone. As discussed previously, the World Health Organization (WHO) informs that there must be an exchange between learners from two or more health professions to constitute this type of learning (World Health Organization [WHO], 2010). Given the silos that exist in health professions education and in clinical practice today, it remains highly unlikely that any two professions can come together to learn without a collaborative effort on the part of their instructors—at the very least to coordinate scheduling. Indeed, the literature on sustaining interprofessional programming stresses empowered collaboration as a means of continued success (Freeth, 2001).

The preceding chapters have outlined the importance of IPE. With two thirds of all sentinel events in the United States stemming from poor communication (Joint Commission, 2007), it seems natural to teach students across professions how to communicate, as well as to equip them with a common language to use when doing so. However, these lessons cannot be ingrained unless students observe and experience them in practice. Similarly, in an educational environment, programming is richer and the benefit to students greater when IPE is generated and presented by instructors modeling collaboration (Interprofessional Education Consortium, 2002). Teaming up to teach about teamwork creates a powerful visual and mental message: there is value to this approach and positive outcomes when employing it.

Engaging other professions in IPE endeavors also ultimately improves the programs themselves. Partnering with representatives from various disciplines helps to maximize the expertise involved in programming and enhances learning by adding the relevant perspectives in both the planning and execution of programs. The Institute of Medicine (IOM) advocates training nurses to "practice to the full extent of their education and training" (Institute of Medicine [IOM], 2010, p. S-1); the impact of many professionals educating together to the fullest of their capabilities is even more powerful, substantially increasing the breadth and depth of teaching experience and information sharing. Furthermore, one profession cannot represent all professions, particularly given distinctive academic and professional cultures. Additionally, as discussed in Chapter 3, current faculty members have not generally been trained in an interprofessional manner, so the collaborative practice (CP) core competencies (Interprofessional Education Collaborative [IPEC] Expert Panel, 2011) do not necessarily feel natural to them.

More simply put, it is practical to enlist the help of others, specifically other disciplines, when implementing interprofessional programming. Clark (2013) outlines the well-documented aforementioned individual cultures of academic disciplines, rife with their own symbols, traditions, and languages. Change is uncomfortable in the best of circumstances, but change without "buy-in" (Kotter, 1995; Kotter and Cohen, 2002)—and especially without knowledge of how to garner such buy-in—can be insurmountable. It becomes necessary to have allies or "insiders" who understand the culture and can help lead culture change on a macro level and interprofessional programming efforts on a micro level. Partnering with those who already speak the language and understand the symbols and traditions can help break down barriers and speed up historically very slow progress, or at least get a foot in the door and a more trusted seat at the table.

Finally, collaboration is a means of ensuring that the needs of all parties involved are met. Expanding accreditation standards around IPE are beginning to result in increased program monitoring and student tracking. Furthermore, increasing pressures to measure the impact of IPE on the Triple Aim—the framework for optimizing healthcare to (a) enhance population health, (b) improve patient satisfaction and outcomes, and (c) decrease costs (Institute for Healthcare Improvement, 2016) are playing a role in directing the nature of IPE programming and evaluation efforts. Collaboration is a way of ensuring these types of programmatic and accountability needs, which are variable by profession, are met. It gives each discipline a voice and also allows for each individual representing those disciplines to speak up about individual needs such as fulfilling team teaching requirements and otherwise receiving recognition for their work (Kezar & Elrod, 2012).

Kezar and Elrod (2012) describe mobilization as the first of three stages of institutional change developing from a study by Kezar and Lester (2009) and the literature (Kezar & Elrod, 2012). During mobilization, preparations for change—recognizing its need, creating a vision, and generating both senior and lateral buy-in—are made. IPE is indeed a change. It is a new way to teach and to learn, which lacks an evidence base as a means of accomplishing the Triple Aim and can be uncomfortable and resisted as unnecessary. The WHO (2010) states definitively that IPE is necessary, asserting that "after almost 50 years of inquiry, there is now sufficient evidence to indicate that IPE enables effective CP, which in turn optimizes health services, strengthens health systems and improves health outcomes" (p. 18). As previous chapters have outlined, although there will be those who steadfastly agree and advocate for IPE even in the face of certain negativism from colleagues and institutional leadership, there will be more who require convincing. This is why mobilization is required.

Even setting aside the potential change and resulting discomfort, faculty members need to be actively mobilized to collaboratively engage in IPE. The aforementioned cultures of academic disciplines create tightly knit communities and can prevent faculty members from fully appreciating the value of interprofessional change (Clark, 2013).

Without widespread and deep understanding of the need for change, as well as in-depth discussions around and shaping of a shared vision and learning goals (Kezar & Elrod, 2012), IPE is often viewed as an "add-on," secondary to other teaching responsibilities and workload obligations. As noted in Chapter 3, to be most effective, the teaching of it necessitates faculty development, which increases the required time commitment involved for those faculty members who will be implementing it. IPE can also be viewed as a competitor for scarce institutional or departmental resources (Kezar & Elrod, 2012), which only increases resistance to it.

Given these barriers to IPE, mobilization may require tangible incentives. Many of the most popular incentives, such as financial compensation, protected time, and inclusion in promotion and tenure decisions, are under the purview of institutional leadership, which is one of many reasons to collaborate from the top down in addition to laterally and from the bottom up. Regardless of any incentive structure, the leadership team needs to support IPE efforts for them to become integrated into the institutional culture, and for collaboration to realize its value. It is not always an easy road, but it is an important one, which begins by identifying and engaging those who can best lead and sustain the agenda.

GETTING STARTED: ASSEMBLING THE TEAM

It is easy to state that IPE cannot be done alone and more difficult to determine who should be involved in the efforts and, importantly, how to get them involved. The literature around implementing and sustaining IPE is clear in its assertion that senior leadership must buy into these efforts for them to persist (Freeth, 2001; Reeves, Goldman, & Oandasan, 2007). There are too many roadblocks, both cultural and logistical, for such programming to survive without support from those who have the power to help diminish or abolish them. Having those on board with access to the resources required to really support IPE and the authority to embed it into the culture and programming is the difference between success and failure. The symbolism alone of backing from the highest levels is very powerful, but from a practical standpoint, making the dean of the school of nursing and other key deans and leaders aware of and ideally getting their support for interprofessional programming will make the journey possible, since at the very least these efforts take time, and any release time required will need the endorsement of senior leaders. More substantially, since IPE requires significant change, which is challenging to push forward without buy-in at all levels, it is particularly important to include those from above.

Although senior leadership is key, the power of localized "champions" cannot be understated (Freeth, 2001, p. 38). These are the faculty whose passion lends intrinsic motivation to drive and support these efforts, sometimes singlehandedly. Their belief in IPE can be infectious, inspiring others and overcoming certain resistance. Aside from serving as a source of inspiration, these are the individuals who provide insight into other professional and discipline-specific cultures and help to advocate and implement change from the inside. They can assist with pushing IPE efforts through their own respective curriculum committees. They are also the faculty and staff members who will be in the trenches, tirelessly working to develop and implement programs at all costs.

Although any initiation of IPE must include the recruitment of individual champions across the various professions involved, IPE should not (and cannot) depend solely on their participation. The burden of champions can be a heavy one, so burnout is to be expected, and turnover in the form of changing institutions, retirement, or death can cause difficulty for the sustainment of IPE without a broader distribution of responsibility (Clark, 2013; Freeth, 2001). Ideally, IPE champions' efforts are compensated from the outset financially, with protected faculty time or through the promotion and tenure process. Recognizing their work in these ways not only helps to retain them and maintain energy and commitment but also demonstrates an institutional (or departmental) commitment to IPE that, again, is symbolically powerful. However, such formal recognition from leadership is not always possible, in which case it is important to find other ways to appreciate the contributions of those who collaborate by example and serve as agents of change for IPE. Lead faculty members spending time to creatively compensate those who support and facilitate activities can make a substantial difference, as long-standing research shows that acknowledgment and appreciation tend to speak much louder than fiscal rewards (Labor Relations Institute of New York, 1946). This could be in the form of recognition at campus events or in institutional publications (Kezar & Elrod, 2012). Even a simple thank-you note or small token of appreciation is sufficient to generate good will and buy-in from those whose support is most needed. These alternative means of compensation will not be enough to ensure long-term sustained success of IPE for the reasons noted earlier and because lead faculty cannot continuously bear such a financial and time-consuming burden; however, they will likely make an important difference in the short run. They may also be sufficient for maintaining the engagement of supporters through the point of becoming champions, perhaps eliminating the need for more formal rewards.

Given the weight that IPE champions bear and the challenge with long-term sustainment of their efforts, it is important to identify other supporters and facilitators in addition to a core group of those most passionate about IPE. This is what Kezar and Elrod (2012) call the *critical mass* of supporters (Mobilization section, para. 10). They are the faculty and staff who are open to change and support IPE on the front lines. They may not be the ones spearheading change or spreading a vision for IPE to colleagues, but they understand its value and help to lead and facilitate IPE activities. Their willingness to support IPE is critical for implementation (Kezar & Elrod, 2012), and their role modeling and work to embed IPE into their own teaching and professional practice are essential for sustainment (Freeth, 2001).

Students, the final group to engage in IPE planning and execution, are discussed in detail in the previous chapter. It is important to reiterate that they are an integral part of any educational program, and their role in planning IPE in particular is invaluable. Much like faculty and staff champions, student champions play a critical part in shaping appropriate programming and encouraging and inspiring their peers, helping to overcome any student resistance. Student support also ensures that programming meets the actual real-time needs of students in addition to the accreditation requirements of the programs in which they are enrolled.

Student participation in both the planning and implementation stages is accompanied by its own set of challenges, however. There are many institutions that simply do not train an interprofessional mix of students and thus have a lack of faculty, staff, students, and other resources to aid in the planning and execution of IPE endeavors.

In these cases, it might be beneficial to collaborate with local institutions that offer complementary programs or, as mentioned in Chapter 7, with community organizations. Mobilizers and organizers are encouraged to think outside the box when seeking partners; no program should be considered inappropriate, and even those outside of healthcare, such as law and business, add significant value to the team. This chapter will later detail the successful partnership between nursing and radiologic sciences at Thomas Jefferson University as an example of how unexpected partnerships can be highly beneficial educationally.

Even those institutions with a plethora of professions represented cannot easily develop programs encompassing several or all of them. In fact, as mentioned in Chapter 4, one of the greatest challenges in IPE is scheduling. Oftentimes schools within the same institution have different academic calendars, but even on the same calendar, the various programmatic structures and formats make scheduling a unique and expansive roadblock. Recognizing this challenge in the initial planning stages and establishing shared time, even courses, during which IPE can take place, will help to make execution feasible. The more embedded it is in the curriculum, the more likely IPE is to be sustained (Freeth, 2001).

The final hurdle to contend with when engaging students in IPE is the students themselves. Whereas some easily see the value of learning one another's roles and collaborating educationally and professionally, eagerly participating in whatever is required of and/or offered to them, others are not so easily convinced. Peer student champions like those described in detail in Chapter 4 can help to encourage the engagement of the latter group, but this will not guarantee attendance at optional IPE activities. Ideally, since students are increasingly overburdened while completing their education and training, they are required to engage in IPE as part of the curriculum. Requiring IPE will ensure that they actually get exposure to it and will also be symbolically significant in indicating the importance of IPE, the core competencies for CP (IPEC Expert Panel, 2011), and team-based practice to the institution and each profession trained there. Otherwise, students may need further encouragement from faculty role models to participate in optional IPE. Additionally, particularly with the rise of accelerated 1-year nursing programs, which leave little time for extracurricular activities, introducing students to IPE early in their programs of study will help to ingrain the value of interprofessional communication and teamwork from a particularly impressionable stage of training. It will also catch students at a time in their training when many simply have more time to devote to optional activities. This is not the case with all health professions programs of study, or even with every nursing program, but for some, the first year often affords the most time for exploration outside of their own curriculum and profession.

ZOOMING IN: GETTING STARTED IN PRACTICE

Thus far, the discussion has centered largely around mobilization and organization of IPE on a macro, or institutional, level. This is important, and as previously indicated, Freeth (2001) informs that those activities which do not become integrated into conventional practice generally do not survive. However, it seems important to also address the assembly of the appropriate team to initiate any one activity to give a sense of mobilization and organization in practice and of a specific process that might be followed.

The organization of an IPE activity begins with a planning team generally composed of individuals representing each profession that will participate in the activity. It is critical for each profession to be represented, as scheduling, format, and desired competency attainment is likely to vary across programs and buy-in is needed from all. Everyone involved need not be a champion, but for the implementation of any new activity, some are needed to push it forward unless the demand for the new activity is coming from senior leadership. Those present in the planning stages must have an idea of their profession's curriculum and IPE accreditation requirements, and ideally they are familiar with the Interprofessional Education Collaborative (IPEC) Core Competencies for Collaborative Practice (Speakman, 2015; IPEC Expert Panel, 2011). This not only will ensure more information sharing and productivity but also will help to maximize learning and core competency attainment for all professions involved.

If the activity is to take place within the curriculum, the planning team will include lead faculty members and perhaps course directors and department heads. An interprofessional committee or center can aid in identifying the appropriate professions to include and faculty to represent them. Without this support, course directors and department heads or deans can help to identify the appropriate leaders, ideally with sanctioned released time to assist. If the activity is to be extracurricular, deans and department heads can assist with identifying facilitators and supporters. It is particularly important to engage departmental and school leadership if the IPE activity will not be embedded in the curriculum, as faculty do not want to create undue and undesirable perceptions about how they are using their protected credit hours. Finally, as noted previously, incorporating students into the planning team is a way to disseminate the rationale and get broader buy-in from learners, as well as to protect their increasingly crowded schedules.

If additional support is needed to conduct the IPE activity after the planning team has outlined it, the group must then recruit additional volunteers. In such instances, it makes sense to seek out the participation of those representing the professions pertaining to the activity being planned. This is often, but not always, the same professions represented on the planning team, which is advantageous from a recruitment standpoint. An example of an activity that would necessitate additional recruitment is an interactive, interprofessional panel to help illuminate a particular case study. Such an activity is described in more detail later in this chapter, but in this case, the planning team would recruit panelists who might actually play a role in the case selected. For an obstetrics unit, for example, the panel could include those from nursing, medicine, pharmacy, physical therapy, and social work, with the panelists each defining their role and responsibilities and explaining their approach to the particular case so that it is framed for students from multiple perspectives.

Once the appropriate professions pertaining to the activity have been identified, the planning committee is left to either consult with an interprofessional committee or center or to perform grassroots efforts to recruit and organize the participants. Either way, recruitment will need to be conducted through in-person, phone, and email contact, and it will require some detailed explanation of the planned activity and student populations involved. It may also necessitate an explanation of what IPE is and why there is a need for it. Some prospective volunteers may need to seek permission to participate from managers or deans, and some faculty development may be required. Furthermore, as discussed previously, since it is difficult to sustain IPE based solely on ongoing volunteer participation, it may be necessary for the planning committee to find ways to creatively compensate, or simply explicitly appreciate, the contributions of any volunteers. Such mobilization efforts connect back to the outset of this section, which focuses on how to get the appropriate individuals at the table to successfully execute IPE.

Getting started can sometimes be the biggest hurdle to implementing IPE, as it can feel overwhelming given the challenges involved. What follows is a guide for initiating culture change, since IPE requires this, and for identifying the appropriate settings and opportunities for IPE. There are numerous challenges that will be addressed as well, but there are also time-tested best practices and extensive literature to support strategies for success.

CREATING A CULTURE OF COLLABORATION

The idea of interprofessional teamwork as a clinical practice approach to promote client-centered care and care transitions is certainly not new. The Association of Rehabilitation Nurses, for example, describes how the healthcare specialty of rehabilitation (rehab) is premised on interprofessional collaboration, which developed in response to the devastating injuries incurred by service men and women in the wars during the 20th century (Association of Rehabilitation Nurses [ARN], 2015). One of the five rehabilitative and restorative principles of rehabilitation nursing necessitates CP to return patients to a maximum level of independence and function within and despite their level of illness or injury (ARN, 2015).

However, what is relatively new is the growing number of proponents of IPE for all healthcare professions in response to the profound changes in the healthcare system of this nation (Bouchaud, 2011; Bouchaud & Gurenlian, 2013; Clark, 2004). The literature is beginning to proliferate with articles supporting the need for and proposed models and evidence-based support of interprofessional collaboration, teamwork, and inclusion of patients as the center of all plans and delivery of care. Educators and administrators of academic institutions and health professions programs are expeditiously redesigning curricula that will prepare new clinicians in their respective disciplines to work together as a team with members from all healthcare disciplines. Academic, clinical, simulation, immersion, service-learning, and experiential opportunities will serve as the settings for these interprofessional healthcare student teams to practice implementing this "new" team approach in all healthcare settings and specialty areas of healthcare practice.

Even with this evidence-based support, and the historical and current practice of rehabilitation supporting the need for and success of interprofessional teams in improving patient outcomes, there remains continued resistance to IPE. Achieving these changes in clinical practice, and more profoundly in the educational preparation of new and future healthcare providers, requires a culture change in both clinical and educational organizations.

As in rehab, the acuity level and complexity of health needs of today's patients who are hospitalized require the attention and coordination of more than one discipline to address their healthcare issues (Bridges, Davidson, Odegard, Maki, and Tomkowiak, 2011; Lumague et al., 2008). The IOM Committee on Quality of Health Care in America (IOM, 2001) recommended an interprofessional approach to address these complex and challenging healthcare needs of the 21st century. The committee suggested that healthcare professionals work in interprofessional teams to achieve a common goal of restoring or maintaining (much like in rehab) an individual's health and improving outcomes. This would be accomplished by maximizing the expertise and perspectives of each of the disciplines through a collaborative team approach (IOM, 2001; Bridges et al., 2011). "The interdisciplinary education of health professionals in the USA has increasingly been tied to renewed efforts directed toward quality improvement in the healthcare system, where problems with communication, collaboration, and cooperation are seen as endemic" (Clark, 2004, p. 251).

However, as noted earlier in this chapter, as well as in Chapter 3, most healthcare providers have been and continue to be educated in silos, within their own profession, and are rarely trained to work as members of, or to be able to lead, integrated teams (Robert Wood Johnson [RWJ] Foundation Health Policy Snapshot Workforce, 2011). What is most ironic about this continued educational approach to preparing healthcare professionals is that from the moment students begin their clinical practicums—almost exclusively in hospital-centric environments—they need to interact with providers from other professions to provide competent, safe, and quality patient care (RWJ Foundation, 2011).

According to Houle and Fleece (2011), we have entered a new time that they refer to as the "New Health Age" (p. 1), which is reflective of transformational changes occurring in healthcare that have been unprecedented and unparalleled in human history. They insist that there is urgency in the need to "create the opportunity for dramatic success and triumph over out-of-control, ever escalating costs and a downward spiral of the health of Americans" (Houle & Fleece, 2011, p. 3). They predict that one third of all hospitals will close by 2020 in response to the shift of healthcare out of acute care settings and into "alternate inpatient settings, ambulatory settings, the home and the community" (Cardillo, 2013, para. 4), as dictated by the consumer, payer sources, and most recently the healthcare reform, or 2010 Affordable Care Act (ACA).

Historically, "preponderant influences affecting nursing education systems and the healthcare organizations in which nurses practice, arise from the practical needs of the current health system, contemporary healthcare issues, and funding and reimbursement availability" (Bouchaud & Gurenlian, 2013, p. 2; Feenstra, 2000; Stanhope & Lancaster, 2006). Accrediting bodies for health professions education programs and healthcare facilities, professional organizations such as the WHO, the American Public Health Association (APHA), the Robert Wood Johnson Foundation, the IOM, consumers, third-party payers, the Triple Aim, and the ACA have been responsible for providing the impetus for IPE of health professionals and transforming academic health centers (Clark, 2004; IOM, 2003).

THE NEED FOR CULTURE CHANGE

Two challenges arise in response to the aforementioned discussion. The first is that, as with rehab, the proposal of an interprofessional team-based approach or interprofessional collaboration between and among the various healthcare disciplines and professionals continues to be a tertiary intervention, which is a continuation of the medical model focused on illness and treatment. This approach is an improved and effective strategy in the *treatment* of patients with the primary aim of *improving* healthcare outcomes. However, healthcare delivery models focused on illness and treatment are inadequate for healthcare workers caring for a population of patients who are presenting with health problems and conditions that persist across decades and/or lifetimes

(Bouchaud, 2011; Maurer & Smith, 2009; Pruitt & Epping-Jordan, 2005; Stanhope & Lancaster, 2006). Today, there is a pressing need to validate IPE and CP as primary intervention strategies for the *prevention* of disease, disability, injury, and premature death.

The second challenge in response to the aforementioned discussion is that of the numerous published articles and professional essentials and recommendations promoting IPE, many have omitted or downplayed the challenges of developing and sustaining these programs in higher education settings (Clark, 2004). Questions around such issues as promoting IPE and collaborative learning in an institution that does not value it or that prioritizes its resources in directions other than IPE programs, securing leadership support in a highly IPE resistive academic environment, and securing institutional and other healthcare disciplinary buy-in arise from the obstacles and challenges impeding the development and sustainability of IPE programs.

Resistance to culture change is to blame for both the failure to fully appreciate interprofessional CP as even a tertiary intervention and the difficulties encountered in initiating and sustaining IPE programs. This resistance to change also accounts for the lack of interest or vision by administrators and educators in considering interprofessional CP as a primary intervention strategy in preventing disease, disability, injury, and premature death. Kotter (1995), recognized as the leading national and international authority on leadership and change, stresses that the number one cause of failure within organizations when attempting to implement change is "not establishing a great enough sense of urgency" (p. 60). The error is that the people involved in the change fail to create for themselves a level of urgency that would entice them to not only take the next step, but to take a step that would challenge them into a new direction (Bouchaud, 2011; Kotter, 2008).

More significantly, Kotter (1995) insists that it is not enough to simply introduce or begin a transformation. Beginning a new program, such as IPE, requires "the aggressive cooperation of many individuals" (p. 60) from all levels of an academic and clinical institution. Without establishing a sense of urgency and need for the IPE program, there is no motivation to invest in it, and "without motivation, people won't help and the effort goes nowhere" (Kotter, 1995, p. 60). In addition, the resistance to change and failure to sustain IPE programs could also result from the fact that initiators and supporters of such programs underestimate just how hard it really is to "drive people out of their comfort zones" (Kotter, 1995, p. 60).

The literature abounds with articles on organizational theories, organizational culture, and theorists and theories on change within organizational settings. The reality is that the addition of IPE and CP requires organizational support, and for many institutions may represent a change in culture. According to Tierney (1988), organizational culture in higher education is a concept that usually does not come up for discussion among the most seasoned of college and university administrators until they find themselves in "moments of frustration, when seemingly rational, well-laid plans have failed or have met with unexpected resistance" (p. 3). He points out that "an organization's culture is reflected in what is done, how it is done, and who is involved in doing it" (Tierney, 1988, p. 3). Academic institutions are also influenced by such powerful external factors as "demographic, economic, and political conditions" (Tierney, 1988, p. 4), and implementing an IPE and CP curriculum is not immune to these factors. "Despite the many benefits and endorsements of IPE and CP, many schools and health systems face numerous barriers to establishing interprofessional programming in a sustainable way" (Speakman, Tagliareni, Sherburne, & Sicks, 2016, p. 10).

When considering change in these academic settings, such as transforming curriculum to include IPE, leaders of this movement must stop to consider that administrators tend to only consider their organization's culture at times of conflict or when adverse relationships ensue. This results in dealing with organizational culture in "an atmosphere of crisis management, instead of reasoned reflection and consensual change" (Tierney, 1988, p. 4). Such a scenario can be seen played out as administrators and department heads of health professions programs are forced to consider fiscal increases, limited resources, and internal and external factors contributing to what feels like another add-on to the curriculum in response to compressed and excelled time frames to meet consumer demands. Therefore, it becomes essential that these leaders in higher education understand their institutions as cultural entities when making decisions related to IPE programs (Tierney, 1988). Concomitant to these institutional barriers is the fact that most nurse and health profession educators are simply ill prepared to develop and lead IPE or CP programming because they themselves have not had formal or experiential training (Speakman & Arenson, 2015).

Clark (2004) concludes that higher educational institutions are "generally inhospitable places for interdisciplinary programs because they are built around vertical structures that tend to differentiate and isolate fields of study rather than to promote a recognition of their similarities and commonalities" (p. 259). He further points out that one needs to also consider the fact that most faculty and administrators were socialized in an environment that encouraged academic specialization and differentiation as they continued along their academic journey of their doctoral degree, promotion, and other achievements. This culture is generally reinforced in traditional academic schools and departments, especially when decisions are being made regarding promotion and tenure (Clark, 2004).

Another consideration that Clark (2004) emphasizes is that although external forces, and even the infusion of external resources, can begin the initiation of change in a long-standing academic culture, the real challenge is in trying to maintain and sustain that change. He goes on to say that any educational organization can "look interdisciplinary" (p. 259) over a short or temporary period of time, especially when being funded through grant initiatives. As noted earlier, to succeed in an academic institution embedded in a well-established culture of tradition and across multiple departments and health education programs, to get that true buy-in from all disciplines over the long term beyond funding and temporary outside scrutiny, those who are truly committed to IPE "must work on multiple fronts—both top down and bottom up—if they are to see any meaningful and permanent change" (Clark, 2004, pp. 259–260). Clark (2004) goes on to say:

> In this effort, the advocate for interdisciplinary programming must be constantly vigilant in identifying and marshaling resources, creative in building structural coalitions and partnerships, and persistent in keeping alive the vision of what interdisciplinary programming should and can be. (p. 260)

IMPLICATIONS FOR NURSING EDUCATION

The IOM *Future of Nursing* report emphasized the need for nurses to lead healthcare change (IOM, 2010). One of the key messages in this report is a call to action for nursing schools to re-envision nursing education that focuses on a population-based perspective and emerging roles for nurses across the care continuum. This redesign of curriculum, be it for diploma, associate, bachelor, or graduate-level programs, will prepare and enable new nurses to focus their nursing practice on primary and community-based care rather than exclusively on acute, hospital-centric care. In calling for nurses to be prepared for emerging roles across the care continuum, and for educators to provide opportunities for nurses to learn and practice how to lead collaborative improvement efforts, the report also includes a vision of preparing contemporary nurses with different competencies that are no longer limited to technical skills. The nursing skillset has now broadened to include participation in and leadership roles on interprofessional teams, as well as full partnership in the redesign of healthcare and improvement efforts. RNs, now and in the future, regardless of their entry level into practice, need to be competent in recognizing the importance of coordinating care and managing transitions across providers and settings, which requires mastery of interprofessional CP competencies.

As established previously, nursing accreditors are increasingly integrating these skills into their standards and visions, providing leverage for IPE at all levels of education and training. Employers are now responding to these accreditors, as well as consumers and payer sources, by increasingly seeking nurses who have been academically and clinically prepared to practice team-based care with a patient-centered focus. However, many factors impact how decisions are made in nursing educational organizations, especially for those resulting in a culture change. The process of decision making in these organizations regarding curriculum content is directly impacted by societal factors (Bouchaud, 2011; Bouchaud & Gurenlian, 2013; Maurer & Smith, 2009; Stanhope & Lancaster, 2006) such as those noted earlier. But there are also internal environmental factors within organizations that impact the decision-making process of nursing educational organizations and the development and implementation of curriculum. Those internal factors include faculty resistance to change, limited resources and inadequate funding, an already crowded curriculum, inflexibility, territoriality, the articulation of leadership, and group decision-making skills (Bouchaud, 2011; Bouchaud & Gurenlian, 2013; Lahti, 1996; Morgan, 1997).

Another aspect of reviewing decision making regarding curriculum change or revision in nursing educational organizations is to address the faculty's resistance to change. Hull, St. Romain, Alexander, Schaff, and Jones (2001) state that revising a nursing curriculum, such as attempting to incorporate IPE, is a faculty-driven, outcome-directed process that can be challenging and at times an agonizing endeavor. Because this undertaking can be accompanied by such self-oriented faculty behavior as inflexibility, indifference, and territoriality, these authors suggest the need for planned, intentional, and goal-directed approaches when considering an academic program revision. Hull et al. (2001) liken this task to trying to move a cemetery. They pose the question of how to balance the vital need for disruption and change while still respecting the sanctity of pre-existing institutions and ideals (Bouchaud, 2011; Bouchaud & Gurenlian, 2013; Hull et al., 2001).

Contributions to group decision making require collaboration. Collaboration requires the cooperation of everybody on the team, as each contributes his or her expertise and experience to the issue being addressed. Insights from seasoned faculty provide structure and guidance for the group, whereas novice members of the group involved in decision making have limited allegiance to tradition and thus are able to ensure that innovative changes are considered. The contributions of all members can foster new ideas, energy, and enthusiasm needed to generate creative strategies in making decisions regarding curriculum revision to include IPE (Hull et al., 2001). This, coupled with communication, compromise, and negotiation—strategic components in the ongoing process of consensus—helps to build and strengthen those involved in decision making. Consequently, the expectation is that all members will receive acknowledgment upon completion of the project (Bouchaud, 2011; Bouchaud & Gurenlian, 2013; Hull et al., 2001).

The educational preparation of nurses and the healthcare delivery system have been dominated by an authoritarian and illness-focused approach whereby those with the presumed knowledge and expertise in healthcare have believed that teaching people something, or providing knowledge, will manifest into compliance and changed behavior. However, Kotter (2008) recognized that knowledge is rarely a sufficient catalyst for change. He discovered that most people believe organizational change can occur in three stages: analyzing the situation, thinking really hard about it, and then just changing it (Kotter, 1990). Those who have invested in transforming the preparation of healthcare professionals to include IPE and interprofessional CP can attest that the "just change it" approach is a long uphill battle that is rarely won or sustained.

In Kotter's experience, this three-prong approach to organizational change plays out so that people *see* something that makes them *feel* something that gives them fire to change: *"see-feel-change"* (Kotter & Cohen, 2002, p. 11). As stated previously, Kotter's first change phase is establishing a sense of urgency. For change to happen, the organization as a whole needs to really want it. As described previously, the *buy-in* is needed by those being affected (Kotter, 1995; Kotter & Cohen, 2002). Currently, there is a culture change occurring in society that is necessitating a similar culture change in nursing education to reflect those societal changes (Bouchaud, 2011). For institutions in the business of educating healthcare professionals, particularly RNs, for practice in the 21st century there must be a conveyed *urgency* related to the fact that they *see* healthcare is really changing and that healthcare is moving toward interprofessional collaborative partnerships and practice. This then would necessitate an urgency to develop and implement IPE programs and CP academically and clinically.

AN IDEALIZED CURRICULUM DESIGN THAT INCLUDES INTERPROFESSIONAL EDUCATION

Throughout the chapter thus far, a broad perspective on IPE has been presented. Now, the focus shifts to a more specific consideration of the incorporation of IPE within a nursing program, and more specifically, one college of nursing's commitment to integrating IPE into the redesign of their undergraduate baccalaureate nursing curriculum. As noted previously, for a change in the educational approach to preparing baccalaureate nursing students to occur, it is critical that the literature provide evidence that instills an urgency in baccalaureate nurse educators and administrators (Bouchaud, 2011; Bouchaud & Gurenlian, 2013). This urgency needs to acknowledge the significance of the shifting paradigm of healthcare and the role IPE plays in preparing baccalaureate nursing students for practice in the changing national and global societal and healthcare environments (Bouchaud, 2011).

According to Bouchaud (2011), "Baccalaureate schools of nursing are organizational institutions composed of three distinct cultures:

> An organizational culture that includes the nursing education institution and its affiliation with other healthcare education institutions and the hospital institution.

> A nursing culture which includes the culture of the nursing profession, the nurse educators, and the nursing students.

> A political culture composed of administrators of the nursing school and hospital, the regulatory agencies that establish and enforce educational mandates, and the community/public health resources" (p. 70).

IDENTIFYING ADDITIONAL INTERPROFESSIONAL EDUCATION SETTINGS AND OPPORTUNITIES

As noted throughout this chapter, the reality of implementing an IPE program is easier said than accomplished, even in the presence of faculty and administrative support and program champions. A consistent theme outlined in this book is the fact that one of the most difficult hurdles in implementing team training is trying to orchestrate a scheduled time that works for more than one discipline of students. Collaboration and team building in terms of patient-centered care are often discussed, but what is also needed is collaboration and team building among the various health professions schools to make it feasible in their course scheduling for students to come together for IPE endeavors. Box 5.1 provides an example of how one university addressed this issue.

CONCLUSION

Since nursing is central to the delivery of healthcare, and healthcare providers are now expected to work with patients, families, and communities to provide team-based care, preparing graduates to be members of interprofessional collaborative teams is essential. To accomplish this goal, leaders of educational institutions and clinical sites need to work together in expressing a shared urgency to afford all health professions students opportunities to engage in real-life, simulated, experiential, immersion, and service-learning interprofessional team-building experiences. Nurse educators have to create meaningful IPE and CP learning opportunities so that nursing students are ready and able to meet these current healthcare needs. As described earlier, this endeavor can be challenging, especially when trying to develop curriculum that involves other health professions.

As discussed in the preceding chapter, it is clear that the ability to implement IPE and CP initiatives relies on support from institutional leadership, faculty, and students. Changes in today's healthcare delivery system require a "new paradigm" of care that focuses on health promotion and maintenance rather than on disease, diagnosis, treatment, and cure. Although team-based patient-centered care has been identified as a way to meet these needs, it is also important to note that this change requires a shift in healthcare and educational culture. As described previously, change is uncomfortable (Kotter, 1995; Kotter & Cohen, 2002), and culture change is particularly difficult when systems have been in place for a significant amount of time. As a result, such change tends to be

BOX 5.1

The Alternative Clinical Experience Day: IVAN©

At Thomas Jefferson University's Jefferson College of Nursing (JCN), an Alternative Clinical Experience (ACE) Day was designed to enhance the completion of a clinical rotation. The students are on campus instead of at their assigned clinical site to conclude their clinical experiences. ACE Day focuses on providing innovative and creative educational opportunities for students to learn a topic or learn about an experience that they might not have encountered during their clinical rotation. Prior to the push for interprofessional education at this university, and prior to the formalized development of the Jefferson Center for Interprofessional Education (JCIPE), the community ACE Day included speakers from various community organizations, politicians, and grassroots committee representatives whose agendas were focused on healthcare issues, and/or lay people who came to speak on topics such as what it is like to live with chronic illness. An ACE Day could include presentations, panel discussions, simulations, case vignettes, group work, and/or videos. In addition, students were given the opportunity to share with each other their clinical experiences and lessons learned during their individual rotations.

However, since partnering with JCIPE, JCN began offering various interprofessional learning experiences on the community ACE Day that have provided nursing students with interactive opportunities to team with radiology students. This partnership has enhanced both student groups' knowledge of the other's role and ability to collaborate with the other profession. It has also positively influenced their understanding of working with patients being discharged from the hospital and with home care patients. The intent of these interprofessional activities is to have the students actualize the impact their joint efforts could have on preventing patients from being hospitalized or at least on decreasing admission and readmission rates, hospital length of stay, and medical errors.

One interactive and effective interprofessional ACE Day teaching strategy involved the use of narrative pedagogy and an unfolding case scenario. The case study—IVAN©, which was based on a faculty member's personal experience—describes a scenario where a patient was poorly managed because of lack of care coordination and interprofessional team collaboration (Speakman et al., 2015).

Initially, nursing and radiology students were placed in team groups and expected to work together to unfold the IVAN© case scenario to a different outcome; they brought their specific discipline experiences and perspectives to the table in a parallel design. To overcome this initial hurdle, the students in each group needed to learn about the other's role. Through interprofessional faculty facilitation, the nursing and radiology students became acquainted and more comfortable coming together as a team. This led to the interprofessional student team members skillfully utilizing their assessment, clinical reasoning, and reflection skills to wed their separate strategies to unfold the case scenario to a different and more positive outcome for the patient, family, and healthcare professionals. Each group then presented their interprofessional practice strategies and projected new healthcare outcomes for this patient case to the class.

During another ACE Day, the IVAN© case scenario was developed into a script, and standardized patients were hired to act out the case study as it originally unfolded and then a second scenario in which a team-based approach was implemented. A class debriefing session followed the two scenarios, focusing on communication, teamwork, and the impact on patient outcomes. Both ACE Days concluded with an interprofessional panel of experts who had been given the same narrative pedagogy and came prepared to present their perspectives on unfolding the case by engaging the students in interactive interprofessional dialogue and role modeling interprofessional collaborative practice exercises. A description of this ACE Day can be found at http://whoeducationguidelines.org/.

Source: Speakman, E., Bouchaud, M., Sicks, S., Giordano, C., & Lyons, K. (2015). FACT ACE Days: Understanding interprofessional approaches to collaborative, patient-centered care. *Transformative Education for Health Professionals.* Available at http://whoeducationguidelines.org

slow and resistance to change high. Schein (2010) describes organizational culture as both dynamic and rigid, the former due to the influence of human behavior that shapes one's values and traditions and the latter as a dimension of one's tendency to set the rules. IPE is continuously evolving, with periods of both dynamic development and rigid resistance.

The final reason to collaborate when mobilizing faculty and administrators and organizing interprofessional programs and activities is for the camaraderie and support collaborators can give. They will make the journey easier, not only by representing and giving insight into different professional cultures but also by sharing in the challenges and rewards of the work. IPE may never quite be done, but celebrating each successful step along the way (Kotter, 1995) helps to continuously renew commitment to the task at hand. Celebrating together enhances both the journey and the shared outcomes, actualizing the commitment to and reality of IPE and collaborative learning environments.

References

Association of Rehabilitation Nurses. (2015). About ARN. Retrieved June 6, 2016, from http://www.rehabnurse.org

Bouchaud, M. (2011). *Preparing baccalaureate nursing students for community/public health nursing: Belief systems and values of nurse educators and administrators.* Ann Arbor, MI: ProQuest LLC.

Bouchaud, M. T., & Gurenlian, J. A. (2013). A qualitative study on preparing baccalaureate nursing students for community/public health nursing as perceived by nurse educators and administrators. *International Journal of Nursing, 2*(2), 43–55.

Bridges, D. R., Davidson, R. A., Odegard, P. S, Maki, I. V., & Tomkowiak, J. (2011). Interprofessional collaboration: Three best practice models of interprofessional education. *Medical Education Online, 16.* Published online April 8, 2011. doi:10.3402/meo.v.16i0.6035

Cardillo, D. (2013). *A new paradigm.* Available at http://www.nurse.com

Clark, P. G. (2004). Institutionalizing interdisciplinary health professions programs in higher education: The implications of one story and two laws. *Journal of Interprofessional Care, 18*(3), 251–261. doi:10.1080/13561820410001731296

Clark, P. G. (2013). Toward a transtheoretical model of interprofessional education: Stages, processes and forces supporting institutional change. *Journal of Interprofessional Care, 27*(1), 43–49. doi:10.3109/1356 1820.2012.730074

Feenstra, C. (2000). Community based and community focused: Nursing education in community health. *Public Health Nursing, 17*(3), 155–159.

Freeth, D. (2001). Sustaining interprofessional collaboration. *Journal of Interprofessional Care, 15*(1), 37–46. doi:10.1080/13561820020022864

Houle, D., & Fleece, J. (2011). *The new health age: The future of health care in America.* Naperville, IL: Sourcebooks.

Hull, E., St. Romain, J. A., Alexander, P., Schaff, S., & Jones, W. (2001). Moving cemeteries: A framework for facilitating curriculum revision. *Nurse Educator, 26*(6), 280–282.

Institute for Healthcare Improvement. (2016). IHI Triple Aim Initiative. Retrieved June 6, 2016, from http://www.ihi.org/engage/initiatives/tripleaim/Pages/default.aspx

Institute of Medicine (2001). *Crossing the quality chasm: A new health system for the 21st century.* Washington, DC: National Academies Press.

Institute of Medicine. (2003). *Academic health centers: Leading change in the 21st century.* Washington, DC: National Academies Press.

Institute of Medicine. (2010). *The future of nursing: Leading change, advancing health.* Washington, DC: National Academies Press.

Interprofessional Education Collaborative Expert Panel. (2011). *Core competencies for interprofessional collaborative practice: Report of an expert panel.* Washington, DC: Interprofessional Education Collaborative. Available at http://www.aacn.nche.edu/education-resources/IPECReport.pdf

Interprofessional Education Consortium. (2002). *Creating, implementing, and sustaining interprofessional education* (Vol. 3). San Francisco: Stuart Foundation. Available at http://matrixoutcomesmodel.com/MatrixFiles/stuart/Volume3.pdf

Joint Commission. (2007). *Improving America's hospitals: The Joint Commission's annual report on quality and safety.* Retrieved June 6, 2016, from http://www.jointcommission.org/assets/1/6/2007_annual_report.pdf

Kezar, A., & Elrod, S. (2012). Facilitating interdisciplinary learning: Lessons from Project Kaleidoscope. *Change: The Magazine of Higher Learning.* January-February, 16–25. doi:10.1080/00091383.2012.635999

Kezar, A., & Lester, J. (2009). *Organizing higher education for collaboration.* San Francisco: Jossey-Bass.

Kotter, J. P. (1990). *A force for change: How leadership differs from management.* Boston: Harvard Business Press.

Kotter, J. P. (1995). Leading change: Why transformation efforts fail. *Harvard Business Review,* March-April (Reprint 95204), 59–67.

Kotter, J. P. (2008). *A sense of urgency.* Boston: Harvard Business Press.

Kotter, J. P., & Cohen, D. S. (2002). *Heart of change: Real life stories of how people change their organizations.* Boston: Harvard Business Press.

Labor Relations Institute of New York. (1946). *Foreman facts.* New York: Author.

Lahti, R. K. (1996). *Group decision making within the organization: Can models help?* Denton: Center for the Study of Work Teams (CSWT) Papers, University of North Texas.

Lumague, M., Morgan, A., Mak, D., Hanna, M., Kwong, J., & Cameron, C. (2008). Interprofessional education: The student perspective. *Journal of Interprofessional Care, 20*(3), 246–253.

Maurer, F. A., & Smith, C. M. (2009). *Community/public health nursing practice: Health for families and populations* (4th ed.). St. Louis, MO: Saunders Elsevier.

Morgan, G. (1997). *Imagin-i-zation.* San Francisco: Berrett-Koehler Publishers.

Pruitt, S. D., & Epping-Jordan, J. E. (2005). Preparing the 21st century global healthcare workforce. *British Medical Journal, 330,* 637–639. doi:10.1136/6mj.330.7492.637

Reeves, S., Goldman, J., & Oandasan, I. (2007). Key factors in planning and implementing interprofessional education in health care settings. *Journal of Allied Health, 36*(4), 231–235.

Robert Wood Johnson Foundation Health Policy Snapshot Workforce. (2011). *What can be done to encourage more interprofessional collaboration in health care?* Available at http://www.rwjf.org/healthpolicy

Schein, E. H. (2010). *Organizational culture and leadership* (4th ed.). San Francisco: Jossey-Bass.

Speakman, E. (2015). Interprofessional education and collaborative practice. In D. M. Billings & J. Halstead (Eds), *Teaching in nursing* (5th ed., pp. 186–196). Philadelphia: Elsevier Health.

Speakman, E., & Arenson, C. A. (2015). Going back to the future: What is all the buzz about interprofessional education and collaborative practice? *Nurse Educator, 40*(1), 3–4.

Speakman, E., Tagliareni, E., Sherburne, A., & Sicks, S. (2016). A guide to effective interprofessional education experiences in nursing education. Washington, DC: NLN Press.

Stanhope, M., & Lancaster, J. (2006). *Foundations of nursing in the community: A community-oriented practice* (2nd ed.). St. Louis, MO: Mosby Elsevier.

Tierney, W. G. (1988). Organizational culture in higher education: Defining the essentials. *Journal of Higher Education, 59*(1), 2–21.

World Health Organization. (2010). *Framework for action on interprofessional education and collaborative practice.* Geneva, Switzerland: Author. Available at http://apps.who.int/iris/bitstream/10665/70185/1/WHO_HRH_HPN_10.3_eng.pdf

6

Creating Experiential Interprofessional Opportunities

Elena M. Umland, PharmD, BS

Julia M. Ward, PhD, RN

As outlined in previous chapters, interprofessional education (IPE) occurs "when students from two or more disciplines learn about, from and with each other to enable effective collaboration and improve health outcomes" (World Health Organization [WHO], 2010, p. 7). Embedded within this definition are levels of learning that result in different outcomes ranging from modification of perceptions and attitudes toward other healthcare professionals and collaborative practice (CP) to improvements in health or well-being as experienced by the patient (Barr, Koppel, Reeves, Hammick, & Freeth, 2005; Reeves, Boet, Zierler, & Kitto, 2015). See Table 6.1.

Collaboration is the key to successful interprofessional healthcare. Interprofessional CP is defined as that which occurs "when multiple health workers from different professional backgrounds work together with patients, families, carers and communities to deliver the highest quality of care" (WHO, 2010, p. 7). It makes sense, then, that the greatest opportunity for ultimately achieving CP exists when students work together in clinical practice, where relationships can be formed and the need for the unique skills of each member is readily evident. Further, the World Health Organization (WHO) acknowledges that the available body of evidence supports the assertion that effective IPE facilitates the achievement of interprofessional CP. To achieve the highest levels of IPE outcomes, changes in behaviors, and changes in overall practice (see Table 6.1, Levels 3, 4a, and 4b), it seems clear that IPE must occur in the clinical, experiential setting. Training healthcare students in this way, in the clinical setting, has the best chance of changing behavior and processes to those that are truly collaborative and will assist the current healthcare system in achieving the Institute for Healthcare Improvement's Triple Aim of improving health outcomes, reducing per capita costs, and improving the patient experience, inclusive of both quality and satisfaction (Institute for Healthcare Improvement [IHI], 2016).

Two broad sets of skills have been identified as necessary for the achievement of collaborative teamwork. Healthcare students must achieve both relational competencies and risk communication competencies (Coulter & Collins, 2011; Fulmer & Gaines, 2014; Legare et al., 2013). Relational competencies include active listening, negotiated agenda setting and prioritizing, demonstration of empathy and emotional intelligence, facilitating involvement, clarification of decisions, values and preferences, and supporting

TABLE 6.1

Outcomes Typology for Interprofessional Education (Barr et al., 2005)

Level 1	Reaction	Learner's views on the experience
Level 2a	Modification of attitudes/perceptions	Changes between groups; changes in perception or attitude toward the value/use of a team approach
Level 2b	Acquisition of knowledge/skills	Includes knowledge/skills related to inter-professional collaboration
Level 3	Behavioral change	Transfer of interprofessional learning to the practice setting
Level 4a	Change in organizational practice	Changes within the organization and delivery of care
Level 4b	Benefits to patients/clients	Improvements in health or well-being of patients/clients

deliberation. Evidence awareness, the communication of risks and benefits, discussion of uncertainties, and the use of decision aids are examples of risk communication competencies (Fulmer & Gaines, 2014).

These two sets of skills can be achieved when students are given the opportunity to practice them (Dwamena et al., 2012; Fulmer & Gaines, 2014); experiential interprofessional opportunities (EIOs) provide these opportunities. Such assertions are validated by research, noting that the most powerful IPE experiences for healthcare students are those that are authentic (Loversidge & Demb, 2014). The definition of authentic includes experiences that are "real," that are noncontrived, and require team collaboration to solve patient problems. In such situations, students resolve to make meaningful contributions to teamwork, as they can clearly see the potential results of failure—notably, negative patient consequences.

STUDENT INVOLVEMENT IN EXPERIENTIAL INTERPROFESSIONAL OPPORTUNITIES

Ultimately, students are incorporated in EIOs to improve healthcare upon their entry into practice; thus, assisting in meeting the Triple Aim. To achieve this, it is anticipated that throughout their IPE experiences, students will need to meet the Interprofessional Education Collaborative (IPEC) Core Competencies (Interprofessional Education Collaborative [IPEC] Expert Panel, 2011) deemed necessary to practice collaboratively.

Early research suggests that EIOs benefit both patients and students (Towle et al., 2010). Students report higher satisfaction working directly with patients and show increased sensitivity to chronic illness, disabilities, mental illness, senior care, and caregiver burden. Further, patients report that they enjoy the companionship of students and feel that their experiences benefit subsequent patients and healthcare providers. One could also argue that EIOs may positively impact the patient experience arm of the Triple Aim.

CREATING EXPERIENTIAL INTERPROFESSIONAL OPPORTUNITIES

Creative EIOs are necessary to produce healthcare student graduates who are practice ready and poised to collectively and collaboratively address the Triple Aim (Institute of Medicine [IOM], 2015). Similar to the creation of any IPE experiences, creating EIOs in the current educational system is challenged with finding the time and ability to schedule the activity. However, the difference and possible advantage of EIOs is that these learning opportunities are created where students practice, and hence where they are already located. The key element is "transforming" those experiences into clinical experiences with learning objectives that includes the IPEC Core Competencies, described in detail in Chapter 2, as well as the relational and risk communication competencies skills noted earlier.

To successfully create these opportunities, faculty and key personnel from each of the programs and/or disciplines that will be involved in the EIO must be "at the table" and take an active role in the development, execution, and assessment (Fulmer & Gaines, 2014). A review of healthcare team training programs found that team training has a positive impact on collaborative team behavior and on care processes (highest outcomes to be achieved with IPE) that ultimately lead to better outcomes for patients (Weaver, Dy, & Rosen, 2014).

EXPERIENTIAL INTERPROFESSIONAL OPPORTUNITIES

Clinical Rounding

Rounding is a term described in the healthcare setting as a meeting of intra- or interprofessionals who gather to discuss patient care plans, provide teaching opportunities for those in attendance, and perform surveillance of patient status at the bedside (Gurses & Xiao, 2006). Bedside rounding particularly has a long history dating back to the early 20th century, when intraprofessional medical or surgical teams stood around a patient's bed and discussed diagnoses and treatments. However, toward the end of the century, rounding more frequently occurred in a conference room instead of at the patient bedside, a practice that caused a breakdown in communication among health professionals and resulted in less than optimal patient experiences (Gonzalo, Chuang, Huang, & Smith, 2010).

Responding to the recent recommendations of several regulating bodies (U.S. Department of Health and Human Services [HHS], 2010; Joint Commission, 2016), interprofessional bedside rounding has been reestablished as a strategy to improve the quality and safety of patient care and to promote positive patient experiences. Furthermore, this reestablished practice has provided health professions students the opportunity to round together with practicing members of an interprofessional group. At Thomas Jefferson University (TJU), bedside rounding was already in place (in situ) and occurred on a regular basis with the surgical team. Students from nursing and then pharmacy were able to join the surgical team and experience firsthand the opportunity to actively participate in the clinical rounding experience while meeting several of the IPEC Core Competencies (see Box 6.1).

Utilizing In Situ Teams as Interprofessional Team-Based Models

The rehabilitation setting has a history of using the team conferencing model as a forum for discussing patients and their disposition (Behm & Gray, 2012). Members of the

BOX 6.1

Clinical Rounding Exemplar

Clinical rounding can be established with two or more student groups. At Thomas Jefferson University, the first established clinical rounding experiences (CREs) included only medical and nursing students rotating through the same medical-surgical service. Pharmacy students were then added along with physical therapy students, who were located off-site and served in a consultant capacity. In the morning, the medical and nursing student assigned to a specific patient met and reviewed the patient's current plan of care, diagnostic and lab study results, and interprofessional plans for discharge. Pharmacy and physical therapy students were encouraged to join the team on-site or to participate remotely via Google Docs® (an online word processing system that allows for the creation of text documents while collaborating with other people in real time). To protect patient health information, no identifying personal information was included on the Google Doc. During the day prior to the rounds with the attending physician, students from each profession would review and add any data or offer any needed consultation. In the afternoon, the students in the health professions who collaborated would present and discuss with the interprofessional team the patient plan of care, and each student answered questions and offered his or her professional assessment. Following the discussion, members directly involved with the patient (medical physician, nurse, and interprofessional students) performed a bedside round that included the patient and/or family to incorporate them as members of the team. Once rounding was completed, students were able to debrief on the experience. Examples of student debriefing statements included the following: *"Communication was a critical skill needed to participate successfully on an interprofessional team"*; *"Collaboration among healthcare professionals was important during the rounding experience"*; and *"Knowing how to interact and listen to other members of the team without using a condescending tone was essential"* (Lyons et al., 2013). Additionally, students who participated in the CRE reported a high level of satisfaction as a team member, experienced increased self-confidence in clinical conversations, expressed a better understanding of each other's roles, and recognized the value of interprofessional input to the patient care plan.

interdisciplinary team are critical to successful patient rehabilitation and are necessary for identifying and providing services to this population of patients that facilitate positive outcomes (Strasser, Uomoto, & Smits, 2008). The model of team conferencing used in the rehabilitation setting today dates back to WWII, when it became necessary to address the needs of the soldiers who survived the war with complex injuries. Although medical advances in surgery and pharmaceuticals facilitated the soldiers' reentry into society, a mechanism to orchestrate and maintain their movement toward sustainability was needed. The team approach with members from a variety of professions was the solution. At TJU, Discharge Disposition Dilemma and Rehabilitation Team Conferences were already in place (in situ) and occurred on a regular basis (Thomas Jefferson University, 2016). Students were then able to join these teams and learn firsthand how interprofessional clinical teams provide patient-centered team-based care (see Boxes 6.2 and 6.3).

Patient Safety and Quality Programs as an Interprofessional Team-Based Model

As in rehabilitation, various inpatient and outpatient settings host safety and quality programs as a way to mitigate sentinel events. For example, the elderly are particularly

BOX 6.2

Discharge Disposition Dilemma Exemplar

The clinical setting generally has already formed in situ interprofessional teams that students can join and participate in as a member of the team. At Thomas Jefferson University, Discharge Disposition Dilemma (DDD) is a team approach to solving a dilemma about a patient's discharge from rehabilitation. The interprofessional team presents a particularly challenging case and engages other clinicians and students in a discussion about potential options and solutions. The student can then observe and subsequently interact with various health professions and observe the dynamics of the clinical team decision making. The students evaluated the teamwork that they observed during the DDD experience and noted that they had a better understanding about the roles and responsibilities of the other disciplines, and by hearing the reasoning from other disciplines, it helped them guide their own practices.

susceptible to falls. In fact, falls in the elderly are a source of significant morbidity and loss of life, as well as an economic burden on the healthcare system. The risk factors for falls are varied in nature and include the presence of certain disease states, the use of certain medications, unsteady gait, immobility, and poor nutritional status. As such, the need for input from a variety of team members to affect any modifiable risk factors is clear (Banez et al., 2008). The success of interprofessional falls prevention programs in delivering patient-centered care with positive patient outcomes has been established (Banez et al., 2008). IPE workshops for health professions students focusing on the clinical skills of occupational therapy, physiatry, and medicine have also been effectively described (Boardman, Al-Jawad, Briggs, & Kendrick, 2010). The implementation of

BOX 6.3

Rehabilitation Team Conference

Typically, members of the rehabilitation team include those individuals who are relevant to the patient's short-term and long-term rehabilitation. At Thomas Jefferson University, the rehabilitation conferencing occurs twice weekly, every Tuesday and Thursday. The team that is meeting usually includes health professionals from medicine, nursing, occupational therapy, pharmacy, physical therapy, and social work. A program manager facilitates the team conference and records student attendance. The program manager is also available to answer any questions raised by students, and during these meetings, students can observe and see a real-time inpatient team conference in an acute rehabilitation setting. After the program manager briefly introduces the conference, students witness how the interprofessional team draws on the expertise of representatives present during the meeting. The team discusses each patient's treatment plan, short- and long-term goals, current status, and plan for discharge. The students observe both discussions about new admissions as well as progress reports for patients who are admitted for longer periods of time, and students gain a sense of the role that insurance coverage plays for patients in this acute rehabilitation setting. At the conclusion of the team meeting, a debriefing session follows, and students have the opportunity to ask questions and clarify any points of confusion. The students evaluate this experience highly and noted that the team of experienced professionals were supporting every aspect of each patient's recovery on the unit and engaged in an open communication, asking questions and assessing the patient as a team (http://www.jefferson.edu/university/interprofessional_education.html).

BOX 6.4

The Falls Assessment Exemplar

Following a provider's referral to the Falls program, a patient would meet with individual members of a team. During this time, they were evaluated via a thorough physical exam and assessments geared toward identifying fall risk, mental status, balance, medication history/adherence, gait, and nutritional status, among others. At the conclusion of the session, and after all of the clinical team had a chance to examine and review the patient's pertinent information, the clinical team would collaborate together to develop an individualized care plan based on the patient's self-identified problems and goals. This was an excellent opportunity for students, depending on the stage in their educational program, to observe and/or participate in this team-based activity. Students could see the specific healthcare roles that are necessary in providing the best care for the patient and observe how the team functions. Student workshops that illustrate the clinical skills needed and the importance of interprofessional teams in addressing falls in the elderly have resulted in improved student understanding of the multifactorial nature of falls, as well as the importance of teamwork by a variety of disciplines to impact falls in the elderly (Boardman et al., 2010).

---

a falls assessment program that includes the patient and/or his or her caregiver(s) as a member, the center of the team, as well as other members of a clinical team, is an example of how a team approach to high-risk vulnerable populations could be effective. The purpose of including this wide variety of practitioners is to address the multifactorial causes of falls in the elderly and to create a care plan that improves the patient's quality of life and can reduce the potential economic burden on the healthcare system; it thus does exhibit a model for addressing the Triple Aim in healthcare. Banez et al. (2008) noted that patient satisfaction was high after implementation of a falls prevention program, and at 3- and 6-month follow-up, persistent improvements in balance, strength, functional mobility, and fear of falling were noted (see Box 6.4).

Teach-back is another example of an interprofessional quality and safety program. It has been determined that low literacy levels impact the ability of patients to interact with healthcare professionals, follow medication instructions, and obtain follow-up care (Dickens & Piano, 2013; Jager & Wynia, 2012). These literacy levels are not often visible to healthcare providers, so it is emphasized that a *universal precaution* be implemented in all healthcare communications and to begin this education during their training programs (Institute of Medicine [IOM], 2003a, 2003b, 2004). In addition, the Office of Disease Prevention and Health Promotion developed the *National Action Plan to Improve Health Literacy* report (HHS, 2010) to address the health literacy problem. A key step in improving health literacy is to educate the healthcare professional about what health literacy is and its impact on patient safety and patient-centered care, as well as the best techniques to provide patient-centered education to these populations. One of these techniques is called *teach-back.*

Using the teach-back technique, patients are asked to explain in their own words what their healthcare provider has told them about their condition and treatment plan. Teach-back allows the healthcare professional to determine if patients understand the information that they have been given. If patients have not attained understanding, it is the responsibility of the healthcare professional to reteach the information in a different

---

BOX 6.5

Nursing-Pharmacy Teach-Back Exemplar

Using the teach-back technique, students from nursing and pharmacy paired together are able to identify a patient who needs additional patient education regarding his or her medication regime and/or side effect warnings. A nursing faculty member, a pharmacy faculty member, a pharmacist, and a nurse provided guidance to the student pair. Both nursing and pharmacy students received formal instruction on the teach-back technique, health literacy, and obtaining a health history prior to their clinical rotation. Student pairs participating in teach-back were assigned selected patients based on the clinical site. After reviewing the assessment data in a virtual team huddle via Google Docs, nursing student participants conducted an oral health history with the selected patients, assessing the patient's health history, health literacy, and learning needs. The nursing student then relayed all findings to the pharmacy student participants via Google Docs. The student team then discussed the morning's findings in person with the nursing clinical faculty and pharmacist before gathering the appropriate teaching materials and meeting with the patient. In this patient meeting, student participants applied the teach-back technique until the patient had demonstrated an understanding of the medication regime. Following the tech-back session, a debriefing with the nursing and pharmacy student focused on health literacy and collaborative patient care techniques.

---

way and to ask the patients to explain in their own words, again, what they have been taught. This process is repeated until patient education and understanding has been attained (Osborne, 2013). See Box 6.5.

IMPLICATIONS FOR NURSING EDUCATION

The nursing credentialing bodies have established that interprofessional experiences should be a part of nursing curricula (American Association of Colleges of Nursing [AACN], 2008; National League for Nursing Commission for Nursing Education Accreditation, 2015). Advancement of nursing education can only be achieved through a revised curriculum that includes EIOs. As mentioned previously, the *Future of Nursing* report (IOM, 2010) called for the transformation of the healthcare system into one that incorporates a team of inter-professionals to collaborate and coordinate patient care. As part of efforts to position nurses as an integral part of the interprofessional team, nurse educators must find ways to prepare students at the undergraduate level by providing experiences that focus on interprofessional communication and collaboration.

The American Association of Colleges of Nursing's *Essentials of Baccalaureate Education for Professional Nursing Practice* (AACN, 2008) requires nurse educators to teach nursing students to "be focused on developing and refining the knowledge and skills necessary to manage care as part of an interprofessional team" (p. 5). The document devotes "Essential VI: Interprofessional Communication and Collaboration for Improving Patient Health Outcomes" to interprofessional experiences alone and maintains that opportunities to develop and enhance interprofessional communication and collaboration will go a long way toward the future delivery of high-quality and safe patient care. Subsequently, the National League for Nursing (NLN) Commission on Nursing Education

Accreditation (2015) "Standard V: Culture of Learning and Diversity—Curriculum and Evaluation Processes" describes the six integrated concepts of the 2010 Education Competency model to include context and environment, knowledge and science, personal and professional development, quality and safety, relationship-centered care, and teamwork (www.nln.org).

Historically, faculty and institutional leadership relied on the early Institute of Medicine reports in 1999, 2001, and 2003, which challenged all health professions to establish curricula that produced clinicians who can practice within an interprofessional team and collaborate to provide safe, quality, patient-centered care to promote the IPE curriculum. Today, considering that all health profession accreditations have included standards about IPE and practice, creating collaborative learning opportunities seems to be in everyone's best interest. Therefore, the need to provide students with opportunities to practice effective communication and learn to collaborate is imperative to create a healthcare environment that naturally provides patient-centered care. Interprofessional clinical opportunities enable baccalaureate graduates to enter the workplace with foundational competencies in communicating and collaborating with members of the healthcare team in ways that improve patient outcomes. EIOs afford nursing students the core competencies identified in the IPEC Expert Panel (2011) report: values/ethics, communication, teams and teamwork, and role and responsibilities. Several interprofessional organizations developed the report, and their input encouraged health professions schools to incorporate the core competencies within their curricula and develop opportunities that best illustrate each one.

In the practice setting, legislation and credentialing bodies also support the establishment of interprofessional teams to ensure the healthcare quality and safety of patients under their care. The American Nurses Credentialing Center [ANCC] (2008), a subsidiary of the American Nurses Association, developed the Magnet® model, which includes a component of exemplary professional practice advocating that nurses should practice within an interprofessional team to promote a positive impact on patient care and outcomes. The Patient Protection and Affordable Care Act (2010) maintains that interprofessional teams must work in a collaborative decision-making process to ensure patient-centered care, thereby improving the quality of healthcare delivery. Nurse educators who prepare nursing students for future practice must keep current legislation and mandates in mind when providing interprofessional opportunities for their students.

CONCLUSION

This chapter supported a 1932 commentary called *Teamwork Within the Hospital*. In that commentary, Rogers asserted that "teamwork is a game played by skilled practitioners, each member fulfilling his post with skill precision to play the game for glory of the game itself" (Rogers, 1932, p. 657). This analogy still holds true and can be applied to today's professional nurses, who play the interprofessional game for the ultimate goal of patient-centered quality and safe care. Clearly, experiences that involve students from a variety of healthcare professions in a clinical setting are beneficial to all—students and patients alike. Challenges do exist, and sometimes barriers to the activity exist, such as a limit on the number of students able to participate given the physical space. However, this should not be a deterrent to moving forward with establishing and maintaining interprofessional experiences for our future healthcare practitioners. By incorporating EIOs within curricula, schools and colleges of nursing are able to meet the core competencies established by IPEC and respond to the educational and practitioner-level credentialing bodies regarding the requirement of developing health professionals who deliver patient-centered care within a team for best outcomes. Moreover, experiential interprofessional opportunities can improve a nursing student's ability to provide optimal care to patients and come to understand how individual plans of care are impacted by CP.

If the ultimate measurement of effective CP is its impact on the Triple Aim (IHI, 2016), then the time is now to create learning opportunities for students to prepare them for team-based models in practice. In Chapter 7, an exemplar of a CP model that is showing great promise in addressing the Triple Aim outcomes is described, but the reality is that this practice model is not a standardized norm integrated in all U.S. healthcare education. "The culture of change that is needed to achieve a closer linkage between education and practice in a collaborative, interprofessional environment will require leadership, careful planning, innovative uses of technology, new partnerships, and faculty development" (Thibault, 2013, p. 1932).

References

American Association of Colleges of Nursing. (2008). *The essentials of baccalaureate education for professional nursing practice.* Washington, DC: Author.

American Nurses Credentialing Center. (2008). *Magnet recognition program application manual.* Silver Spring, MD: Author.

Banez, C., Tully, S., Amaral, L., Kwan, D., Kung, A., Mak, K., et al. (2008). Development, implementation, and evaluation of an interprofessional falls prevention program for older adults. *Journal of the American Geriatric Society, 56*(8), 1549–1555.

Barr, H., Koppel, I., Reeves, S., Hammick, M., & Freeth D. (2005). *Effective interprofessional education: Argument, assumption and evidence.* Promoting Partnership for Health Series. Malden, MA: Blackwell.

Behm, J., & Gray, N. (2012). Interdisciplinary rehabilitation team. In K. L. Mauk (Ed.), *Rehabilitation nursing: A contemporary approach to practice* (pp. 51–62). Sudbury, MA: Jones & Bartlett.

Boardman, K., Al-Jawad, M., Briggs, L., & Kendrick, D. (2010). Falls assessment and prevention: A multidisciplinary teaching intervention. *Clinical Teacher, 7*(3), 206–210.

Coulter, A., & Collins, A. (2011). *Making shared decision-making a reality.* London: King's Fund.

Dickens, C., & Piano, M. R. (2013). Health literacy and nursing: An update. *American Journal of Nursing, 113*(6), 52–57. doi:10.1097.01.NAJ.0000431271.83277.2f

Dwamena, F., Holmes-Rovner, M., Gaulden, C.M., Jorgenson, S., Sadigh, G., Sikorskii, A., et al. (2012). Interventions for providers to promote a patient-centred approach in clinical consultations. *Cochrane Database Systematic Reviews, 12*, CD003267. PubMed PMID: 23235595

Fulmer, T., & Gaines, M. (2014). *Partnering with patients, families, and communities to link interprofessional practice and education.* New York: Josiah Macy Jr. Foundation.

Gonzalo, J. D., Chuang, C. H., Huang, G., & Smith, C. (2010). The return of bedside rounds: An educational intervention. *Journal of General Internal Medicine, 25*(8), 792–798. doi:10.1007/s11606-010-13

Gurses, A., & Xiao, Y. (2006). A systematic review of the literature on multidisciplinary rounds to design information technology. *Journal of the American Medicine Information Association, 13*(3), 267–276. doi:10.1197/jamia.M1992

Institute for Healthcare Improvement. (2016). IHI Triple Aim Initiative. Retrieved June 7, 2016, from http://www.ihi.org/engage/initiatives/tripleaim/Pages/default.aspx

Institute of Medicine. (2003a). *Health professions education: A bridge to quality.* Washington, DC: National Academies Press. Available at http://www.nap.edu/catalog/10681.html

Institute of Medicine. (2003b). *Keeping patients safe: Transforming the work environment of nurses.* Washington, DC: National Academies Press. Available at http://www.nap.edu/catalog/10851.html

Institute of Medicine. (2004). *Health literacy: A prescription to end confusion.* Washington, DC: National Academies Press. Available at http://www.nap.edu/catalog/10883.html

Institute of Medicine. (2010). *The future of nursing: Leading change, advancing health.* Washington, DC: National Academies Press.

Institute of Medicine. (2015). *Measuring the impact of interprofessional education on collaborative practice and patient outcomes.* Washington, DC: National Academies Press.

Interprofessional Education Collaborative Expert Panel. (2011). *Core competencies for interprofessional collaborative practice: Report of an expert panel.* Washington, DC: Interprofessional Education Collaborative.

Jager, A. J., & Wynia, M. K. (2012). Who gets a teach-back? Patient-reported incidence of experiencing a teach-back. *Journal of Health Communication: International Perspectives, 17*(Suppl. 3), 294–302. doi:10.1080/10810730.2012.712624

Joint Commission. (2016). Hospital: 2012 National Patient Safety Goals. Retrieved June 7, 2016, from http://www.jointcommission.org/the_joint_commission_launches_campaign_to_reduce_readmissions/

Legare, F., Moumjid-Ferdjaoui, N., Drolet, R., Stacey, D., Harter, M., Bastian, H., et al. (2013). Core competencies for shared decision making training programs: Insights from an international, interdisciplinary working group. *Journal of Continuing Education in the Health Professions, 33*(4), 267–273. PubMed PMID: 24347105

Loversidge, J., & Demb, A. (2014). Faculty perceptions of key factors in interprofessional education. *J Interprof Care, 29*(4), 298–304. doi: 10.3109/13561820.2014.991912.

Lyons, K. J., Giordano, C., Speakman, E., Isenberg, G., Antony, R., Hanson-Zalot, M., et al. (2013). Jefferson interprofessional clinical rounding project: An innovative approach to patient care. *Journal of Interprofessional Care, 42*(4), 197–201.

National League for Nursing Commission for Nursing Education Accreditation. (2015). NLN CNEA accreditation. Available at http://www.nln.org

Osborne, H. (2013). *Health literacy from a to z: Practical ways to communicate your health message.* Burlington, MA: Jones & Bartlett Learning.

Patient Protection and Affordable Care Act. (2010). 42 U.S.C. § 18001 et seq.

Reeves, S., Boet, S., Zierler, B., & Kitto, S. (2015). Interprofessional Education and Practice Guide No. 3: Evaluating interprofessional education. *Journal of Interprofessional Care, 29*(4), 305–312. doi:10.3109/13561820.2014.1003637

Rogers, D. (1932). Teamwork within the hospital. *American Journal of Nursing, 32*(6), 657–659.

Strasser, D. C., Uomoto, J. M., & Smits, S. J. (2008). The interdisciplinary team and polytrauma rehabilitation: Prescription for partnership. *Archives of Physical Medicine and Rehabilitation, 89*(1), 179–181. doi:10.1016/j

Thibault, G. (2013). Reforming health professions education will require culture change and closer ties between classroom and practice. *Health Affairs, 32*(11), 1928–1932.

Thomas Jefferson University. (2016). Rehabilitation team conferences. Available at http://www.jefferson.edu/university/interprofessional_education.html

Towle, A., Bainbridge, L., Godolphin, W., Katz, A., Kline, C., Lown, B., et al. (2010). Active patient involvement in the education of health professionals. *Medical Education, 44*(1), 64–74.

U.S. Department of Health and Human Services, Office of Disease Prevention and

Health Promotion. (2010). *National action plan to improve health literacy.* Washington, DC: Author.

Weaver, S. J., Dy, S. M., & Rosen, M. A. (2014). Team-training in healthcare: A narrative synthesis of the literature. *BMJ Quality and Safety, 23*(5), 359–372. PubMed PMID: 24501181

World Health Organization, Department of Human Resources for Health. (2010). Health Professions Network Nursing and Midwifery Office within the Department of Human Resources—a framework for action on interprofessional education and collaborative practice. Available at http://www.who.int/hrh/nursing_midwifery/en/

7

Community-Based Interprofessional Education: Partnerships Promoting Health and Well-Being

Karen T. Pardue, PhD, RN, CNE, ANEF
Shelley Cohen Konrad, PhD, LCSW, FNAP
Jennifer Morton, DNP, MPH
Trisha A. Mason, MA

Interprofessional education (IPE) and collaborative practice (CP) have gained significant attention in the acute care arena for improving patient care outcomes. In larger schools of nursing with ready access to academic medical centers, these approaches to care delivery are often realized through medical, surgical, special care unit, and emergency department clinical rotations. Academic medical centers provide opportunity for diverse health professions faculty and students to come together to learn with, from, and about each other for improving collaborative approaches to care (Angelini, 2011).

Yet many nurse educators do not work in educational settings aligned with an academic medical center. In-patient acute care represents services targeted at the individual level; to transform the U.S. healthcare system, the focus needs to shift to improving the health of populations (Institute for Healthcare Improvement, 2016). The Patient Protection and Affordable Care Act (ACA) seeks to ensure accessible, cost-effective, and high-quality care for all (Patient Protection and Affordable Care Act, 2010). A community-based approach captures everyday practice, reflecting naturalistic settings where people live and work within their own communities.

Community-based IPE provides an alternate rich learning opportunity for faculty and students, and one that is readily translatable for nurse educators. It is not uncommon for nurses to be already engaged in promoting health and providing care in the community. Such care provision has historically been broad in form, ranging from services targeting vulnerable underserved populations to advocating for culturally diverse communities to facilitating the patient/family transition from hospital to home. These collective activities are complex, revealing the need for an interprofessional collaborative approach to support optimal population-based outcomes (De Los Santos, McFarlin, & Martin, 2014).

BUILDING A MODEL FOR COMMUNITY-BASED INTERPROFESSIONAL EDUCATION AND PRACTICE

While acute care environments are commonly advanced for learning interprofessional collaboration, community-based settings provide a real-world context for developing teamwork and communication skills. Students are eager to learn through hands-on experiences, such as those provided through public health activities, service-learning, and preclinical and clinical educational opportunities (Bridges, Davidson, Odegard, Maki, & Tomkowiak, 2011; Hettinger & Gwozdek, 2015; Lee, Hayes, McConnell, & Henry, 2013). Care delivery in community settings cultivates cross-professional communication, teamwork for shared patient-centered problem solving, and enhancement of disciplinary role understanding (Bridges et al., 2011; Interprofessional Education Collaborative [IPEC], 2011). Additionally, these natural environments foster new awareness and behaviors with respect to cultural humility, health literacy, relational connection, and resourcefulness. Such behaviors generalize across team roles and are relevantly applied in community-based work with diverse individuals, populations, and life circumstances (Adams, Orchard, Houghton, & Ogrin, 2014; Bridges et al., 2011).

The Interprofessional Community Model (ICM) for Community-Based Interprofessional Education and Practice describes four conceptual dimensions essential for collaborative community-based learning: Infrastructure/Support, Student Learning Outcomes, Community as Partner, and IPE by Design (Figure 7.1). These dimensions are inextricably linked and rely on one another for building successful interprofessional programming.

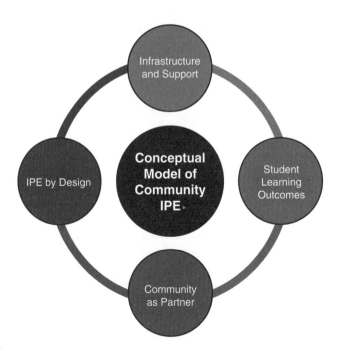

FIGURE 7.1 The ICM (2015) Model for Community-Based Interprofessional Education and Practice. (Copyright © Karen T. Pardue, 2015.)

Infrastructure and Support

Creating an interprofessional culture for learning depends on institutional, departmental, and individual engagement (Bridges et al., 2011; Oandasan & Reeves, 2005b). Community-based IPE begins with faculty vision, passion, and creativity. As noted previously, IPE endeavors must have committed faculty champions; this is particularly important in all population-based endeavors, as these leaders tout the benefits of collaborative learning and embrace experiences that positively impact the health and well-being for their community of interest. Departmental support through systematic dialogue within and across academic programs cultivates a culture of collaboration. Cross-departmental communication is facilitated through intentional and regularly scheduled meetings, rendering an opportunity for faculty to exchange ideas and integrate IPE across professions. This paradoxically systematized yet organic process fosters cohesion among the faculty and engenders a culture characterized by genuine communication, teamwork, and the cocreation of learning. Institutional resources that support a culture of interprofessionalism include but are not limited to allocation of time for interprofessional pursuits, value for team-based faculty scholarship, support for faculty development, and the forging and maintaining relationships with external partners (Barnsteiner, Disch, Hall, Mayer, & Moore, 2007; Bridges et al., 2011; Oandasan & Reeves, 2005b).

Student Learning Outcomes

In establishing beneficial student learning outcomes, the institutional core values need to align with the core competencies delineated by the report of the Interprofessional Education Collaborative (IPEC) Expert Panel (2011). Collaboration, leadership, critical thinking, compassion, and health and wellness guide all educational programming and community-based activities identified in the exemplars in this chapter. In combination, these values and competencies inform the development of student learning outcomes for community-based, interprofessional learning experiences. The IPEC Expert Panel report is a useful reference for faculty in developing cross-disciplinary learning outcomes (Pardue, 2015).

As outlined previously, to ensure meaningful student learning outcomes that advance the curricular imperatives for individual programs, it is optimal for IPE activities to be codeveloped by faculty from participating departments. Codevelopment also provides opportunities for faculty to work with each other to fill curricular gaps that otherwise might not have been met. For example, community-based interprofessional learning commonly highlights threads addressing health disparities and cultural perspectives that all programs need to fulfill their accreditation mandates (Cohen Konrad & Browning, 2012). This approach is echoed by Villarruel, Bigelow, and Alvarez (2014), who specifically challenge nurse educators to experientially integrate the 3Ds—diversity, disparities, and social determinants of health—into clinical education. Through such engagement, students learn firsthand about the exigencies of low resources, lack of access, cultural barriers, and disparities in care. Community-based IPE experiences cultivate critical reflection, compassion, social justice, and civic responsibility, rendering rich educational outcomes.

Community as Partner

Community-based IPE/collaboration and the partnerships inherent within them should not be left to chance. All too often, health education is situated in traditional paradigms that regard professionals as serving the community rather than viewing health as an interactive and collaborative process. These conventional approaches, although altruistic in nature, may actually be ill informed and harmful to the populations that they are attempting to serve. In addition to the benefits outlined in Chapter 4, including community partners as informants to health curricula and as full members of the education team ensures culturally relevant teaching and learning. Exposure to diverse health perspectives and practices adds to students' knowledge of contextual and cultural differences (Morton, 2012). Therefore, this model's inclusion of committed community partners expands faculty and students' capacity to learn with and from the community and practice in low-resourced, population-based settings (Airhihenbuwa, 2007).

Academic and community-based partnerships are reliant on shared trust and common commitments. Trust is established in this dyadic relationship through active listening and mutual respect, and compromise is often needed to realize distinctive organizational goals. The focus for academic institutions commonly centers on meeting students, educational requirements, and for the community, it is often to address a community want or need; the synergy of the partnership emerges in the compromise to achieve both.

Moreover, establishing community-based trust means an assurance of a longitudinal presence and commitment to the programs while maintaining ongoing dialogue and process evaluation that leads to refinements. It is also critical that partnerships are built and maintained with the understanding that each other's needs are met through interventions that are of low burden for all stakeholders involved.

Interprofessional Education by Design

As described earlier, simply creating a colocation is not sufficient for true interprofessional learning—interaction is required. Although students from different disciplines attending a lecture exemplify a cross-professional audience, true interprofessional learning requires dialogue among participants and, at best, an active shared experience (D'Eon, 2004; Oandasan & Reeves, 2005a). Like building community partnerships, interprofessional learning should not be left to chance (Pardue, 2013). In community settings, this means that interprofessional service-learning and other community-based shared opportunities are framed by IPEC Core Competencies and also are intentionally facilitated using interprofessional pedagogical methods. Without clear objectives, active teaching strategies, and intentional direction, students and faculty gravitate to their own disciplines, reluctant to engage with others. Hence, students learn best when they observe their faculty engaged in interprofessional teaching and modeling collaboration in real time with their faculty colleagues (Pardue, 2015).

THE UNIVERSITY OF NEW ENGLAND: A CASE STUDY OF COMMUNITY PARTNERSHIPS AND INTERPROFESSIONAL EDUCATION

The University of New England (UNE), a health science university grounded in the liberal arts, is organized around six different colleges: the College of Arts and Sciences, the

College of Osteopathic Medicine, the College of Dental Medicine, the College of Pharmacy, the College of Graduate and Professional Studies (online programming), and the Westbrook College of Health Professions. This unique institutional focus on health professions preparation provides an ideal environment for advancing IPE and CP. In collaboration with collegiate administration (Pardue), the director of the IPEC and the School of Social Work (Cohen Konrad), the director of nursing (Morton), and the coordinator for service learning (Mason), faculty from diverse disciplines and departments are engaged in interprofessional endeavors and champion a culture of collaborative learning and practice. The university does not house an academic medical center, resulting in clinical education dispersed across health delivery systems throughout the state of Maine, with select programs maintaining practice sites throughout the country. Strong clinical relationships are essential for translating campus-based IPE into the actual care of patients.

There is substantial and inherent value in community-based clinical education. Working with populations across the life span with diverse backgrounds and cultures supports learning outcomes applicable to all health profession disciplines and provides an ideal context for collaborative learning and practice. In addition, the ever-changing healthcare environment has created a mandate for new clinical education paradigms. A community-based interprofessional clinical experience is one way to accomplish this call for reform. At UNE, before any community exposure takes place, faculty and students actively engage in cultural preparedness training in concert with our community partners. This includes exercises in self-reflection and identity, as well as an exploration of one's own biases in the context of the community of interest. The following exemplars illustrate the use of this model in conceptualizing, implementing, and evaluating community-based IPE experiences. Table 7.1 summarizes the exemplars that are described in Boxes 7.1 through 7.3.

IMPLICATIONS FOR NURSING EDUCATION

It is undoubtedly challenging to prepare students for a healthcare world that has yet to fully take shape. As discussed previously, the implementation of the ACA, with a goal of increasing access for millions of previously uninsured people, renders a time of substantial reform in healthcare delivery. Systems thinking, improved coordination of care, and a focus on health promotion are essential tenets in this healthcare redesign, and nursing as a profession plays a key role. Nursing has a rich tradition of coordinating care services and has long recognized the impact of community and environment on individual, family, and community health. Nurse educators are therefore uniquely poised to advance the integration of community-based IPE into clinical curricula. How might this be achieved?

At the macro level, nursing faculty can look to several professional organizations for leadership and guidance in preparing students to meet the needs of diverse communities and an ever-changing care delivery system. The National League for Nursing (NLN), through publication of the 2015–2016 *Public Policy Agenda,* acknowledges the complexities of today's healthcare delivery and identifies the priorities of access, education, diversity, and workforce in addressing this challenge. Through enhancing access, this blueprint for governmental action advocates for community education and wellness services, highlighting the parallel need for nursing education to prepare

Text continued on page 87.

TABLE 7.1

Framework for Community-Based Interprofessional Education

Element → Program ↓	Infrastructure & Support	Student Learning Outcomes	Community as Partner	IPE Design
Touchstone Foundation	UNE administration UNE faculty and students from dental hygiene, nursing, physician assistant, physical therapy, pharmacy, and social work Office of Service Learning	Use unique and complementary abilities of all team members to optimize patient care (IPEC, 2011, p. 21). Develop a trusting relationship with patients, families, and other team members (IPEC, 2011, p. 19).	Touchstone staff Touchstone administration HOME Team ride-alongs Local community substance abuse service agencies Touchstone clientele	Planned orientation Training to address the vulnerability of this population Student-designed health promotion activities Reflective writing exercises
Community Health Fairs	UNE administration UNE faculty and students as noted earlier UNE dental hygiene clinic Office of Service Learning In-kind supplies	Explain the roles and responsibilities of other care providers and how the team works together to provide care (PEC, 2011, p. 21). Communicate with team members to clarify each member's responsibility in a treatment plan or public health intervention (IPEC, 2011, p. 21).	Community leaders representing various aggregates: elders, pediatric population, immigrant/refugee groups, targeted locale or neighborhoods City health officials Church/faith leaders Community agencies and service resources	Prefair orientation Education addressing best practices for screening Event navigators Student-designed health screenings and education Concepts of culture, health literacy, and age-appropriate teaching Session debriefing
Riverside Medicine Institute (RMI)	UNE administration UNE faculty and students from medicine and pharmacy Faculty from UNE IPEC Josiah Macy Jr. Foundation funding	Engage other health professionals (appropriate to the situation) in shared patient-centered problem solving (IPEC, 2011, p. 25). Organize and communicate information with patients, families, and the healthcare team in a form that is understandable (IPEC, 2011, p. 23).	RMI administration RMI clinicians RMI patients with complex comorbidities at risk for rehospitalization	Faculty and student orientation Modified TeamSTEPPS® training Shared patient panels in ambulatory clinic Shared home visits Shared didactics Case study presentation Reflective journals

BOX 7.1

Touchstone Foundation Interprofessional Community Experience

The Touchstone Foundation (anonymized) provides emergency shelter, meals, laundry, and shower facilities to homeless men struggling with drug and alcohol dependence. The 41-bed shelter facility is colocated with an onsite 16-bed coed inpatient detoxification program. The site is medically managed and hosts a staff of nurses, doctors, and caseworkers supporting its mission to help those struggling to overcome addiction.

Additionally, Touchstone offers an innovative community outreach and support program—the Homeless Outreach and Mobile Engagement (HOME) Team. This team collaborates with municipal officials and the downtown business alliance to engage individuals who may be exhibiting disruptive or unsafe behaviors. HOME team members provide a safe, friendly, and familiar helping hand to those with chronic mental health and substance abuse issues who are living on the streets. Team members educate and encourage client participation in needed social services while providing a cost savings to the city by reducing law enforcement and emergency medical services.

The service-learning activities at the Touchstone shelter grew out of a successful program at another city shelter, where UNE students from nursing, physician assistant, and pharmacy programs delivered foot soaks and health promotion activities. Upon learning about the positive experiences and interactions between students, faculty, and shelter clients, Touchstone approached the University of New England (UNE) about providing similar services to the population they serve. As the Touchstone clientele is unique, UNE faculty and Touchstone staff joined in thoughtful and careful discussions as to how best implement a program that addressed the needs of clients without being intrusive while simultaneously providing a safe and rich learning environment for students. All parties identified the necessity for an orientation to prepare students (and faculty) regarding the particular health needs and challenges of this population, promote communication and role understanding between students and staff, and examine and share biases and assumptions about working with this population.

At the suggestion of UNE partners, students are additionally afforded an opportunity to shadow the HOME team. Through this mobile van experience, students witness firsthand the collaboration that occurs between Touchstone outreach staff and law enforcement in keeping clients safe. This innovative outreach exemplifies team-based approaches, which respect the dignity of people and help to prepare students for their in-shelter service activities. Student comments from this preparatory experience illustrate the imperative for orientation and preparation:

"Prior to my visit, I probably would have been extremely intimidated by a homeless person. Now, I know they are people living day to day, just trying to survive while their quality of life seems to have no positive outlook. I can only hope that I have as much compassion as the workers of Touchstone to make a positive impact on this population."

"It wasn't until our last trip that I realized I was staring at a man who was just that, a man. He was a person. Even if he lived outside. Even if he was intoxicated. He was a man that needed help."

Conceptualizing the Touchstone experience required open and honest communication between program staff and the UNE Office of Service Learning. It was important to ensure that planned shelter activities be mutually beneficial and worthwhile. A regular and sustained presence is critical to building trust with this community, but at the same time, UNE did not want to overcommit its faculty in providing supervision of these services. Touchstone was balancing uncertainties as well, acknowledging the benefits of a shelter-based health promotion program while voicing uneasiness as to how such programming disrupts established routines. Loss of routine can be quite unsettling

(continued)

BOX 7.1

Touchstone Foundation Interprofessional Community Experience (*continued*)

to select clientele. It was therefore important to consider the appropriate number of students for each session so as to not overwhelm the environment. Furthermore, there was commitment to providing interprofessional student teams the opportunity to work together in shaping activities for this service-learning experience.

Faculty champions emerged from UNE programs of dental hygiene, nursing, physical therapy, physician assistant, pharmacy, and social work. This faculty leadership team met with the service-learning coordinator to determine a menu of services that not only addressed the population needs identified by Touchstone but also fit within their respective scopes of practice. Areas of cross training and scope overlap were also identified so that students could work together and thereby learn about the similarities and differences in their roles. This led to student recognition of specific talents and contributions of the various disciplines:

"I really appreciated having nursing there and how comforting they were towards their patients. They seemed so relaxed and I thought they did a good job. They even made me feel more comfortable."

"Also in small talk it was nice to interact with [each other] as students. We had something in common so it didn't feel forced. We asked for their opinion so that was cool."

Twice per month, interprofessional teams of students provide on-site health promotion. Based on the prior popularity of foot soaks, which illustrated the ease of conversation when clients' feet are bathed in warm water, each session always offered this service. Other examples of health promotion activities include blood pressure screenings, gait analysis, seated stretches and exercises, fluoride varnishes, games, and interactive discussions with clients in the detoxification program.

Evaluation of student learning included a postexperience survey and a reflective writing assignment. Analysis of data revealed that this community-based experience favorably impacted students' attitudes and behaviors for working on an interprofessional team with a vulnerable population:

"I really enjoy the service learning experience at Touchstone. It demonstrates the need in the community and how all professions can contribute to addressing this need. The gentlemen at the shelter show great appreciation for the services and [it] makes you realize the effect we can have."

It was important to continuously listen to UNE partners and adjust programming based on feedback. On some evenings, clients were receptive to a multitude of health promotion offerings, and other times they were less engaged. Touchstone staff, in contrast, consistently accessed the health programming, asking questions, for example, about diabetes management or safe transfer techniques for a wheelchair-bound client. Over time, students' conceptualization of the Touchstone community expanded to include support and administrative staff, thereby recognizing the staff as an integral part of the interprofessional team addressing client safety and well-being.

Another lesson arose as students reexamined their definition of health services. Initially, students were eager to perform hands-on skills, as such activity commonly defines novice learners' perceptions of their discipline. Over time, students and faculty came to understand that performing foot soaks and assessments, although initially not viewed as a health profession skill, provided a desired service and served as an indispensable vehicle for communication, relationship building, and the establishment of trust.

BOX 7.2

The Population-Focused Health Fairs Interprofessional Community Experience

Background

One of the most inclusive ways that the University of New England (UNE) has been able to engage students in interprofessional public health outreach activities is through community health fairs. Working with community representatives and a multitude of stakeholders, health fairs provide valuable win-win partnerships that advance health promotion screening and education, strengthen community access to local resources, and enhance collaboration among local service providers while teaching students teamwork, communication, resourcefulness, and the barriers faced by many in our immediate community. It is useful to target a health fair event to a specific vulnerable population, such as an immigrant or refugee community, a homeless aggregate, a pediatric or older adult population, or a unique neighborhood. This approach supports provision of tailored services and resources to optimally address the health interests and needs of the identified aggregate.

The conceptualization of a health fair reflects a collaborative process. Inclusion of neighborhood leaders, city health officials, faith/religious members, resource providers, faculty, and students ensures that the selected screenings, education, and resources are those most needed and desired by the community. Visibility and engagement of community leaders encourages event turnout and promotes trust with the community of interest. The participation of local providers or referral agencies is important and promotes sustainability of interventions.

The process of designing a health fair provides students from different disciplines the opportunity to work together. Once community needs are identified, roles and responsibilities for various stations can be divided, resulting in enhanced cross-disciplinary communication. Additional education or research may be necessary in planning the event, providing opportunity for peer instruction. Faculty or community representatives can engage with local agencies and resources for their participation in the event. Community leaders can support fair publicity, but this also provides occasion for students in non–health programs, such as business or marketing, to apply their talents in promoting the event.

A comprehensive health fair targeting senior citizens reflects one particular community-based interprofessional education program highlight. This event, sponsored at UNE's campus-based dental hygiene clinic, achieved the multiple goals of providing local seniors access to a variety of health assessments, screenings, and services while simultaneously showcasing a low-barrier oral health clinic. By partnering with the Southern Maine Agency on Aging, city health officials, and an intercultural community center, specific elder health needs and services were identified. Faculty and partners led cross-disciplinary students in a prefair orientation, which included an overview of roles and responsibilities of different professions, referral information, and appropriate teaching considerations for working with elders. During orientation, students were encouraged to be curious about each other, ask questions, and observe how other professions learn about and interact with patients. Students were then assigned to interprofessional teams to facilitate each station, with oversight and mentorship provided by faculty.

Attendees were greeted by event navigators (social work students), who provided information on fair services and available resources. Participants were then guided to a comprehensive dental hygiene station where teams of students were ready to offer a variety of services, such as flu shots (delivered

(continued)

BOX 7.2

The Population-Focused Health Fairs Interprofessional Community Experience (*continued*)

by nursing students), blood pressure screenings (delivered by physician assistant students), diabetic foot checks and prediabetes screenings (delivered by pharmacy students), fall prevention assessments and instruction (delivered by physical therapy students), and oral health screenings and assessments (delivered by dental hygiene students). This collaborative model had students working together as teams in delivering numerous screenings, assessments, and interventions to an individual patient. A debriefing was conducted at the conclusion of the fair to elicit student learning and discoveries. A formalized student evaluation survey revealed the merit and strength of learning about and from cross-disciplinary interaction:

"I enjoyed watching and listening to other students' interactions with the patients. It was interesting to hear students talk about information they have learned in their program."

"[B]eing in a situation that requires interacting with people receiving services while working with people from other professions is valuable to me"

Engaging students and community leaders with one another in health fair planning provides a powerful interprofessional service-learning experience. Through this process, students learn to collaborate with others, listen and receive feedback from team members, share accountability with other disciplines, and apply leadership practices.

Lulls in participant activity were reframed from time wasted to time appreciated, as such breaks rendered opportunity for students to informally talk with one another about their common and discipline-specific responsibilities and practices. For example, students were unaware of dental hygiene's role and scope of practice in health promotion and cancer screening. The hygiene students demonstrated the use of a VELscope®, an adjunctive device used to screen the mouth for neoplasms, bacterial, or fungal infections. Similarly, pharmacy students described and demonstrated the use of a monofilament for diabetic neuropathy screening. Nursing students discussed immunization practices and discovered that pharmacy students share in administration of vaccines. These unanticipated organic and candid student-to-student interactions proved to be invaluable, engendering cross-disciplinary connections that endured over time as students continued to see one another on campus and regard each other as resources in their health professions studies.

The importance of faculty engagement in public health outreach activities is another lesson that was reinforced through the health fairs. Although students enter into service activities with the best of intentions, they need instructive assistance to ensure high-quality outcomes meaningful to the community of interest. Health education is an intervention, and faculty oversight safeguards accurate, culturally congruent, and age-appropriate teaching. Interprofessional health fairs provide many excellent teaching moments that demonstrate real-life examples of doing no harm, the need for appropriate knowledge and referral capabilities should an issue arise in screening, and the ability to clearly understand the limits of delivering care as students. Faculty model interprofessional collaboration and demonstrate best practices to ensure favorable impact of public health outreach and education.

BOX 7.3

The Riverside Medicine Institute Community Experience

The Riverside Medicine Institute (RMI—anonymized) represents the community-based practice arm of a regional hospital. This organization has a long tradition of serving underinsured and uninsured populations, including those living with complex health and mental health conditions. Approximately 32,000 outpatient visits occur each year at RMI, and increasingly, many of these take place in the home with people identified at discharge from acute care as "at risk" for rehospitalization. Nurse practitioners, physicians, physician assistants, medical assistants, and medical residents are based at the site, with pharmacy and social work professionals providing routine care and consultation.

The interprofessional collaborative clinical experience at RMI was envisioned and designed by RMI clinicians and University of New England (UNE) educators. Administrators from both institutions were engaged during the earliest phase of development and kept apprised of its advancements and implementation. A significant and often complicated aspect of developing RMI's interprofessional clinical experience was establishing both external and internal trust. Positive working relationships had to be constructed between the collaborating institutions (nexus) and also across the participating health professions within and across each program. Thus, two monthly meetings took place during the planning year: one with members of both institutions becoming familiar with each other's priorities and practices and the second with each program getting to know each of the participating professionals who would be carrying out the interprofessional clinical experience pilot. Although the development process was lengthy, it ensured that educators would model behaviors that we hoped students would be learning in their clinical experiences.

During conceptualization, the interprofessional clinical experience planning group thoughtfully addressed anticipated scheduling, staffing, curricular, and assessment hurdles. The inaugural clinical experience included students and preceptors from the medical and pharmacy colleges. Clinical site preceptors from those colleges oversaw their students and exposed them to the practices of other professions, such as nurses, medical assistants, and social workers. The selection of only two disciplines was intentional, as starting small, using rapid cycle evaluation, and benefiting from lessons learned supported more enduring program success when additional students were added in the future.

At RMI, interprofessional clinical experiences are woven into the traditional placement through assignments and clinical opportunities. Students share patients 1 day a week doing home and clinic visits, briefing prior to and debriefing following each visit with a clinical preceptor. Students additionally participate in common weekly didactic sessions covering content of shared relevancy, such as diabetes medications and managing patients with mental health and substance abuse disorders. During the course of their 5-week shared clinical experience, students are required to complete three reflective journal entries. Each entry is guided by a prompt that asks students to critically analyze aspects of communication, teamwork, ethical dilemmas, and knowledge of each other's responsibilities as practiced in their community setting.

For the final interprofessional clinical assignment, the pharmacy and medical student pair present a case study. The assignment is carefully designed to integrate content commensurate with single-discipline (medicine/pharmacy) learning outcomes, as well as common interprofessional clinical evaluation measures. Faculty discovered that the assessment tools included clinical objectives that reflected the interprofessional behaviors of communication, teamwork, knowledge of roles and responsibilities, and ethical conduct, and with slight wording changes became generic and thereby useful in evaluating nursing or any student in the health professions.

As outlined in Chapter 3, faculty readiness is essential to the success of interprofessional clinical experiences. UNE provided an interprofessional education orientation session and a modified TeamSTEPPS® training prior to launching the initial pilot. Monthly meetings offered support, direction, and mentorship to preceptors actively engaged with students and also to those playing supportive roles at the site. Preceptors

(continued)

BOX 7.3

The Riverside Medicine Institute Community Experience (*continued*)

described these sessions as especially beneficial in the sense that they understood that although specific disciplines needed to oversee clinical education, any one of them could facilitate learning about communication, teamwork, and patient centeredness—aspects of interprofessional competencies. Knowing this seemed to reduce preceptor stress and increase commitment to the interprofessional clinical pilot.

Similar to previous exemplars in this book, the students participating in the RMI-UNE interprofessional clinical experience are also initially dubious about the value of learning with and from each other through shared rotations. For example, the medical students wonder what they could conceivably learn from pharmacy students, and pharmacy students ponder what they possibly have in common with future physicians. At the conclusion of placements, however, the majority of students describe RMI as a transformational educational experience that positively changed their perceptions of other health professions and emphasized the essentialness of interprofessional team-based care. The words of the following pharmacy student echo the sentiments of the 40-plus students who now yearly flow through RMI's clinical-community education:

"[RMI] gave me an opportunity to see how dependent everyone is on each other in a medical facility. With each of these professionals having various roles and responsibilities, they are all able to work together with a common end goal of providing the utmost care and maintaining the well-being of a patient. Having a collaborative work environment with involvement from different health care professionals allows for a solution to any problem that may arise in a healthcare setting."

The RMI clinical experience is now entering its third year and growing. This site has become a sought-after community placement for pharmacy and medical students. The RMI-UNE faculty meet periodically to revise and improve shared learning assignments and opportunities, as well as to consider ways to grow interprofessional practices in their community-based clinic. The next phase will include social work and nursing students, with other professions to follow.

There are several lessons learned from the original community-based RMI pilot. Many at RMI noted that they have directly profited from the interprofessional clinical experience. For example, practitioners are now systematically conducting more team-based home visits, having witnessed their utility with student learners. Benefits include reduced number of visits with individual practitioners, lowered costs, reduction of medication mishaps that might have led to lessened quality of health for patients and unnecessary visits to the emergency department or primary care practitioner, and patient satisfaction—all of which exemplify Triple Aim goals (Institute for Healthcare Improvement, 2016).

Worries about increased workload due to interprofessional learning have diminished. RMI-UNE educators and administrators understand that setting up placements takes time and intention, but once roles are clearly established and schedules aligned, the clinical learning flow becomes relatively seamless. This is not to minimize the work involved with interprofessional clinical experiences, but rather the lesson learned is that the benefits are worth the extra effort.

Last, as stated earlier, faculty and preceptor readiness, training, and mentorship are essential and ongoing features of interprofessional clinical/community placements. As noted in Chapter 3, faculty need basic knowledge and conceptual buy-in, as well as skills in interprofessional facilitation to create successful learning for students. Students learn best when instructors model interprofessional behaviors and when community sites commit to team-based practices.

The RMI experience provided UNE with opportunity to build a curricular model for interprofessional clinical-community education. With the support of the Josiah Macy Jr. Foundation, UNE's Center for Excellence in Interprofessional Education conducted two interprofessional collaborative practice summits. These gatherings brought together community-based health practices to learn about and from others engaged in changing health professions education and the healthcare practice landscape. UNE now has four additional sites utilizing the interprofessional model, with future plans to expand to rural community settings in the northern region of Maine.

students for such responsibilities. The agenda upholds IPE and CP as a new and innovative approach aimed to improve healthcare delivery and health outcomes (National League for Nursing [NLN], 2015). The NLN's core value of diversity is thoughtfully addressed, highlighting how race/ethnicity, religion, socioeconomic status, age, gender, and geography can adversely influence population health (NLN, 2015). Students therefore need guided experiential education where constructs of social bias, cultural health inequity, and social determinants of health can be explored. Through such experiences, graduates become prepared for real-world practice and can favorably impact the healthcare delivery systems where they will work. This public policy agenda should be reviewed by all nurse educators, with perhaps time dedicated at a faculty meeting to examine the priorities and consider how they can network locally with legislators to advance this agenda.

The American Association of Colleges of Nursing (AACN) provides additional macro-level guidance and leadership in advancing population-based care and IPE. AACN core principles reflect respect and inclusion for diverse opinions, experiences, and cultures, and the organization's vision promotes the contribution of nursing in leading safe, high-quality healthcare systems (American Association of Colleges of Nursing [AACN], 2015). The *Essentials of Baccalaureate Education for Professional Nursing Practice* (AACN, 2008) clearly explicates the requirement for IPE, offering suggestions for curricular content/activities that develop effective communication, teamwork, and collaboration abilities among nursing students.

At an institutional level, nursing faculty, from licensed practical nursing to doctoral preparation, need to consider how to integrate community-based IPE into their programs of study. Applying the framework presented in this chapter may prove helpful. In considering partnerships, one first step might be to connect with a colleague from another department who shares a same commitment for providing experiential learning opportunities where students can practice teamwork and communication in real-life settings. Successful partnerships can also be established with programs outside of traditional healthcare, including psychology, business, and education. Starting small with just one other program provides an opportunity to work through obstacles that arise and supports successful collaboration. Faculty additionally need to cultivate an interest and partnership with a local agency, program, or organization, as such relationship is essential for gaining entry into a community and identifying a population-based interest or gap. Developing both internal and external partnerships requires an investment of time and effort to build mutually open and trusting connections.

There are several structural considerations in the design of community-based IPE. Timely and clear communication with institutional administration, such as a director, dean, or supervisor, reflects an essential facet when forming external partnerships. Administrative awareness and buy-in helps to ensure that appropriate infrastructure, support, and resources are available for community-based IPE learning. Designing the experience itself requires cocreation by faculty (and students) representing the different programs, with leadership and guidance from community partners. Students learn collaborative abilities by working together in collaborative activities, thereby necessitating active pedagogical approaches. Implementation requires consideration as to the nature of the experience, whether curricular or cocurricular, and methods for assessing student learning and population health outcomes.

CONCLUSION

The healthcare challenges that confront our society are growing ever complex, engendering calls for reform of health professions clinical curricula to better reflect today's real-world problems. Nurse educators need to take risks and expand clinical horizons beyond the traditional acute care setting. Service learning provides a value-added experience for students, often outside of or as a complement to their curricular expectations. This teaching strategy engages both students and faculty, together with community partners, in hands-on learning within a real-world setting, often with vulnerable populations. Reciprocity is a hallmark of service learning, whereby students and community partners mutually benefit from cocreating meaningful service, with learning occurring through action and critical reflection (National Youth Leadership Council, 2015). All stakeholders are empowered through shared decision making and thoughtful planning and preparation employing a strengths-based approach that upholds community assets rather than fixing an identified or perceived need (Seifer & Connors, 2007). In this way, service learning fosters leadership, communication, teamwork, cultural humility, and resourcefulness for students beyond the classroom and clinical settings.

Concomitantly, collaborative interprofessional community-based education provides students with firsthand experience as to how coordinated team working, cross-disciplinary knowledge of roles and responsibilities, clear communication, and a patient-centered orientation favorably impacts health outcomes. Additionally, these learning opportunities vividly illustrate the influence that environment, cultural preparedness, and access to appropriate care and resources have on individual and population health and well-being. When students are exposed to and taught interprofessional principles and skills in an integrated, real-world manner, they are more likely to seamlessly transition from learner to professional graduate, fully prepared to contribute to a patient-centered collaborative team-based workforce.

References

Adams, T. L., Orchard, C., Houghton, P., & Ogrin, R. (2014). The metamorphosis of a collaborative team: From creation to operation. *Journal of Interprofessional Care, 28*(4), 339–344. doi:10.3109/13561820.2014.891571

American Association of Colleges of Nursing. (2008). *The essentials of baccalaureate education for professional nursing practice.* Retrieved June 7, 2016, from http://www.aacn.nche.edu/education-resources/BaccEssentials08.pdf

American Association of Colleges of Nursing. (2015). About AACN. Retrieved June 7, 2016, from http://www.aacn.nche.edu/about-aacn

Angelini, D. (2011). Interdisciplinary and interprofessional education. *Journal of Perinatal and Neonatal Nursing, 25*(2), 175–179. doi:10.1097/JPN.0b013e318212ee7e

Airhihenbuwa, C. O. (2007). *Healing our differences: The crisis of global health and the politics of identity.* New York: Rowman & Littlefield.

Barnsteiner, J., Disch, J., Hall, L., Mayer, D., & Moore, S. (2007). Promoting interprofessional education. *Nursing Outlook, 55*(3), 144–150. doi:10.1016/j.outlook.2007.03.003

Bridges, D. R., Davidson, R. A., Odegard, P. S., Maki, I., & Tomkowiak, J. (2011). Interprofessional collaboration: Three best practice models of interprofessional education.

Medical Education Online, 16, e1–e10. doi:10.3402/meo.v16i0.6035

Cohen Konrad, S., & Browning, D. (2012). Relational learning and interprofessional practice: Transforming health education for the 21st century. *Work, 41*(3), 247–251. doi:10.3233/WOR20121295

De Los Santos, M., McFarlin, C., & Martin, L. (2014). Interprofessional education and service learning: A model for the future of health professions education. *Journal of Interprofessional Care, 28*(4), 374–375. doi:10.3109/13561820.2014.889102

D'Eon, M. (2004). A blueprint for interprofessional learning. *Medical Teacher, 26*(7), 604–609.

Hettinger, L., & Gwozdek, A. (2015). Utilizing community-based education as a springboard for interprofessional collaboration. *Access, 29*(3), 10–13.

Interprofessional Education Collaborative Expert Panel. (2011). *Core competencies for interprofessional collaborative practice: Report of an expert panel.* Washington, DC: Interprofessional Education Collaborative.

Institute for Healthcare Improvement. (2016). IHI Triple Aim Initiative. Retrieved June 1, 2016, from http://www.ihi.org/engage/initiatives/tripleaim/Pages/default.aspx

Lee, M. L., Hayes, P. A., McConnell, P., & Henry, R. M. (2013). Students delivering health care to a vulnerable Appalachian population through interprofessional service-learning. *Gerontology and Geriatrics Education, 34*, 43–59. doi:10.1080/02701960.2013.737388

Morton, J. (2012). Transcultural healthcare immersion: A unique interprofessional experience poised to influence collaborative practice in global settings. *Work, 41*(3), 303–312. doi:10.3233/WOR-2012-1297

National League for Nursing. (2015). *Public policy agenda: 2015-2016.* Retrieved June 7, 2016, from http://www.nln.org/docs/default-source/advocacy-public-policy/public-policy-brochure2015-2016.pdf?sfvrsn=0

National Youth Leadership Council. (2015). What is service-learning? Retrieved June 7, 2016, from http://nylc.org/service-learning/

Oandasan, I., & Reeves, S. (2005a). Key elements for interprofessional education: Part 1: The learner, the educator and the learning context. *Journal of Interprofessional Education, 19*(Suppl. 1), 21–38. doi:10.1080/13561820500083550

Oandasan, I., & Reeves, S. (2005b). Key elements for interprofessional education: Part 2: Factors, processes and outcomes. *Journal of Interprofessional Education, 19*(Suppl. 1), 39–48. doi:10.1080/13561820500081703

Pardue, K. T. (2013). Not left to chance: Introducing an undergraduate interprofessional education curriculum. *Journal of Interprofessional Care, 27*(1), 98–100. doi:10.3109/13561820.2012.721815

Pardue, K. T. (2015). A framework for the design, implementation and evaluation of interprofessional education. *Nurse Educator, 40*(1), 10–15. doi:10.1097/NNE.0000000000000093

Patient Protection and Affordable Care Act. (2010). 42 U.S.C. § 18001 et seq.

Seifer, S. D., & Connors, K. (Eds.). (2007). *Faculty Toolkit for Service-Learning in Higher Education.* Scotts Valley, CA: National Service-Learning Clearinghouse. Available at https://ccph.memberclicks.net/assets/Documents/FocusAreas/he_toolkit.pdf

Villarruel, A. M., Bigelow, A., & Alvarez, C. (2014). Integrating the 3D's: A nursing perspective. *Public Health Reports, 129*(Suppl. 2), 37–44.

8

Using Technology to Support Interprofessional Education and Collaborative Practice

Dimitrios Papanagnou, MD, MPH, EdD (c)
Kathryn M. Shaffer, EdD, MSN, RN, CNE

The literature is replete with studies that support technology's ability to foster significant improvements in achieving educational milestones. Used to support both teaching and learning, "technology infuses learning spaces with digital tools; expands course offerings, experiences, and learning materials; supports asynchronous learning; builds 21st-century skills; increases student engagement and motivation; and accelerates learning" (EdTechReview, 2013). Technology has the potential to transform instruction by creating new paradigms for collaboration across professions. Via technological modalities, collaborations are fostered between facilitator and learner, learner to professional content and resources, and learners across varied professions. With its ability to personalize learning, accelerate the rate of learning, and shape learner-to-learner collaborations, educational technology has the untapped potential to redefine interprofessional education (IPE) in the health professions.

IPE is gaining momentum across the country and is embedded in many healthcare professions accrediting bodies. The Commission on Collegiate Nursing Education, *Essentials of Baccalaureate Education for Professional Nursing Practice* (American Association of Colleges of Nursing, 2008), and the Commission for Nursing Education Accreditation (Speakman, 2015) standards address the core knowledge expected of graduates of baccalaureate nursing programs and address interprofessional communication and collaboration as a means to improve patient health outcomes.

With the establishment of focused, IPE-rich curricula, students in the health professions are no longer learning in isolation. Rather, at an early stage in their careers, students are beginning to understand the roles, complexities, and contributions that other professions make to improve patient health outcomes. IPE provides opportunities for students to engage in decision making while focusing on patient-centered care.

The IPE pedagogy is dynamic and complex. As described previously, finding a common strategy for multiple disciplines to agree on can be challenging. Using an educational foundation for IPE, however, can support the type of transformative learning that is essential for making the substantial changes in attitudes and behaviors in students in health professions—particularly those students in the nascent stages of their training. In doing so, changes in the ways health professionals practice will ensue, which will ultimately improve patient outcomes (Oandasan & Reeves, 2005).

It has already been established that the logistics of scheduling students from multiple professions can be a significant barrier to implementing IPE and collaborative practice (CP) learning opportunities. The integration of collaborative technology tools can help bring together students who would not otherwise be able to join interprofessional collaborative educational experiences. Computer-supported collaborative learning (CSCL), for example, is the educational process that provides groups of learners the opportunity to collaboratively construct knowledge on a topic in pursuit of a learning goal or objective with the assistance of a computer (Graesser, Chipman, & King, 2008). This is just one example that highlights a vital trend that has emerged: the importance of technology-assisted learning in fostering IPE in the health professions.

Appropriately preparing students for collaborative practice (CP) necessitates structured learning experiences that include collective problem solving and group interaction, as well as an active learning environment that allows for the transfer of knowledge into practice (Wellmon, Gilin, Knauss, & Linn, 2012; Nisbet, Hendry, Rolls, & Field, 2008). Technology can be used to develop the structured environments needed for students to develop the knowledge, skills, and attitudes of CP.

While providing students with the opportunities to collaborate with others, technology also affords students learning environments that are easy to use, in real time, and collaborative—despite any logistical and scheduling barriers that may present along the way.

TECHNOLOGY IN INTERPROFESSIONAL EDUCATION AND COLLABORATIVE PRACTICE

The past several years has been marked by a technological explosion, as there has been a big push on all fronts to incorporate technology into education. Simply, students expect it and 21st-century skills demand it. It is clear that the use of technology in educational programs creates a milieu of engagement, retention, and critical thinking. Unfortunately, however, some educators are still intimidated by unfamiliar technology. If technology is to be incorporated into education thoughtfully and not perceived as an added burden for educators, how can it be accomplished successfully and seamlessly?

It is conceivable that treating technology as a *pedagogy* will help educators discover which modality works best for their learning environment and students at any given time. A theoretical framework that lends itself for adoption into educational programming, specifically IPE, is Technological Pedagogical Content Knowledge [TPACK] (Koehler & Mishra, 2008; Figure 8.1).

Educators within a particular discipline possess *content knowledge* of what they know and what students need to understand to function in their roles. *Pedagogical knowledge* refers to the ways educators would prefer to have that content be delivered to their students, such as written assignments, reflections, and discussion groups. By comprehending the *content* and *pedagogical knowledge,* the educator can transition to *technological knowledge.* How does the educator successfully use technology to enhance the transformation of content for his or her students while being cognizant of

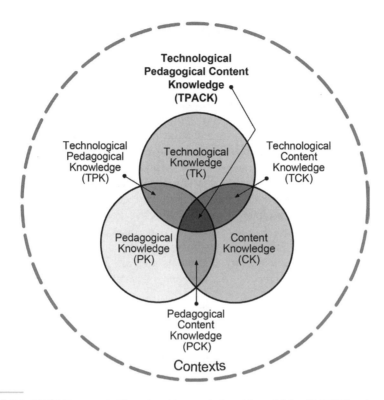

FIGURE 8.1 TPACK Framework. (Reproduced by permission of the publisher © 2012 [tpack.org].)

his or her pedagogical approach? The integration of technology into education offers a thoughtful approach to instruction, as technology should ideally enhance, not take the place of or be an addition to, the educator's approach.

Most educators are familiar with Bloom's taxonomy, a framework to develop higher-order thinking in students. Named after Benjamin Bloom, an educational psychologist, three domains of learning (i.e., cognitive, affective, and psychomotor) are identified to create learning outcomes that can develop critical reasoning skills in students. Bloom theorized that through the cognitive domain (i.e., through the acquisition of knowledge), students could develop their intellectual skills (Bloom, Engelhart, Furst, Hill, & Krathwohl, 1956). From simple to complex, he created a classification system to develop intellectual cognitive ability.

Interestingly, technology has been applied to Bloom's taxonomy to show its practical use in this digital age and to highlight how Bloom's taxonomy can be integrated into e-learning. For instance, the Padagogy Wheel by Allan Carrington (http://tinyurl.com/bloomsblog)—note the spelling to highlight its subtle reference to the iPAD and other tablet devices—categorizes various applications (i.e., apps) that can support higher-order thinking as delineated by Bloom's taxonomy (i.e., remember → create → evaluate → analyze → apply). Another example is Mike Bloom's Visual Bloom's (https://visualblooms.wikispaces.com), which similarly ascribes various technological programs compatible with mobile devices that have the potential to nurture the stages of higher-order thinking in learners.

COMMUNITIES OF PRACTICE AND TECHNOLOGY

Technology can enhance the quality and delivery of the educational content at hand. As discussed previously, IPE focuses on CP, whereby students who learn together are able to create a knowledge-rich environment that helps establish the foundations for evidence-based practices. These knowledge-rich environments display some of the distinct characteristics that social learning theorists term *communities of practice* (CoP) (Shaffer, 2014). CoPs are groups formed to engage in cooperative learning in a common "domain" (Wenger, 1998). They are distinguished from other learning environments based on three key characteristics: domain, community, and practice. Wenger (1998) defines a domain as the group's shared interest. Members of the group are committed to the domain (or interest) but possess a set of shared competencies that distinguish them from others who may share interest in that respective domain. Members within the group (or community) engage in joint activities and social exchanges that help each other both share and gain information. Members interact and learn together. Essentially, the practice is defined by members, who themselves are practitioners in the shared community's interest. Over time, these practitioners develop a shared repository of collaborative resources.

The design framework of Wenger (1998) is applicable in technology-rich IPE and CP learning environments. In this framework, participants work together through activities and reflection, and together they can overcome differences to address specific issues. This framework supports the use of IPE in collaborative learning environments, such as clinical settings. Students who engage in patient-centered care develop an understanding of another individual's expertise and knowledge brought to a healthcare team; this exchange enhances the overall healthcare team and ultimately has the potential to directly impact the quality of care delivered. In addition to further understanding the roles and responsibilities of their own respective profession, students also have the ability to understand how they, themselves, function as part of the healthcare team.

Transitioning from IPE to CP is a current focus of educating students in the health professions. "A consensus is emerging that the healthcare professionals of the future must have the competency to work in teams to provide collaborative care and that their educational experiences should prepare them for this by providing them with robust and meaningful interprofessional educational experiences" (Thibault, 2013, p. 1930).

Technology can play an essential role in supporting CoPs. "Information technologies provide opportunities for CoPs to facilitate communication among members from different geographic locations and time zones, increasing the diversity of the learning network" (Ho et al., 2010, p. 140). In addition, Ho et al. (2010) make the argument that "eCoPs offer theoretical and tangible benefits to health professions who hold disparate expertise" (p. 140).

GENERATIONAL DIFFERENCES AND TECHNOLOGY

Much has been written over the past several years about generational differences across Baby Boomers, Generation X, and Millennials (i.e., Generation Y). It is important, however, to first understand their value systems, interaction styles, and learning preferences to effectively integrate technology into educational contexts. Many, if not most, interprofessional groups in healthcare are composed of multiple generations; therefore, better understanding them will help educators develop highly collaborative functioning teams.

Baby Boomers, born between 1946 and 1964, are optimistic, ambitious, have good communication skills, work efficiently, and are team oriented. They have already acquired many of their technological skills, and the communication style that they prefer is through email and the Internet (WMFC).

Generation X, born between 1965 and 1980, are adaptable, focused, self-starters, and project oriented. They have been assimilated with technology and enjoy the latest technology. They like handheld devices, and their preferred communication style is through email. They are also likely to engage in online media (WMFC).

Millennials (or Generation Y), born between 1981 and 1997, are self-confident, diverse, sociable, innovative, and out-of-the-box thinkers. They are open to new ideas, thrive in collaborative work environments, and generally want to make a difference. They are technologically savvy, as technology has been an integral part of their lives. Millennials expect the technology to be flexible, however, as some are technology dependent. Their preferred communication style is through mobile devices, the Internet, social media, and texting (Coomes & DeBard, 2004).

TECHNOLOGICAL APPLICATION IN INTERPROFESSIONAL EDUCATION AND COLLABORATIVE PRACTICE

It has already been established that today's healthcare environments are using technology to help providers stay connected with their patients. Similarly, this format is being used in health professions education as a way to prepare students for a delivery system that utilizes health information systems. The issue then becomes how to protect patient information in a technology-rich environment. When selecting a technology to use in IPE or CP, faculty must understand the security of that technology and how they can limit the risk of patient personal information from being compromised. Designing activities with de-identifiable information or interaction thorough secure networks will help to limit information exposure. Checking with your institution's HIPAA and technology policy will help to guide your learning opportunities.

Simulation Technology in Interprofessional Education

Although much remains to be learned about the ideal ways to assist learners in understanding interprofessional competencies, simulation-based methodologies have the potential to help model the real-world practice of healthcare, where teamwork often happens asynchronously across time and space (Interprofessional Education and Healthcare Simulation Symposium, 2012). In 2011, the Society for Simulation in Healthcare (SSH) and the National League for Nursing (NLN) identified an opportunity to enhance IPE outcomes by better leveraging the intersection of IPE and healthcare simulation (Interprofessional Education and Healthcare Simulation Symposium, 2012) (Figure 8.2).

With the overarching goal of improving performance, enhancing patient safety and quality, and reducing errors in healthcare, simulation-based methodologies and technologies can provide a safe learning environment. These technologies can take many

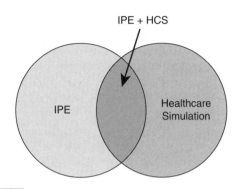

FIGURE 8.2 The Intersection of IPE and Healthcare Simulation (HCS).

forms, including low-fidelity part- and full-task trainers, higher-fidelity patient simulators, virtual reality programs, computer-based simulations, and standardized patients
(Interprofessional Education and Healthcare Simulation Symposium, 2012).

Partial task trainers, or low-technology simulators, are replica (anatomic) models or
manikins for learners to practice and gain competence in simple techniques and/or
procedures; these represent the lowest-fidelity tools in simulation-based education and
may take place independently or in group formats (Decker, Sportsman, Puetz, & Ballinger,
2008). Screen-based computer simulators employ programs that acquire knowledge,
assess competency of knowledge acquisition, and provide feedback related to clinical
knowledge and critical thinking skills (Decker et al., 2008). Virtual reality simulators take the
technology one step further: They combine a computer-generated environment for the
learner, with tactile, auditory, and visual stimuli via partial trainers to promote enhanced
authenticity (Decker et al., 2008). Standardized patients use case studies and role-playing
in a simulated learning experience; typically, paid actors or peer learners are trained to
portray a specific patient presentation in a realistic and consistent manner (Decker et al.,
2008). Full-scale simulators, or medium- to high-fidelity simulators, typically incorporate
a computerized full-body manikin that can be programmed to provide realistic physi-
ologic responses to learners' actions and interventions. Simulations using this technology require a realistic environment and allow for the use and integration of actual medical and/or surgical equipment and supplies (Decker et al., 2008).

Research suggests that two key elements of IPE are addressed by simulation: the
opportunity to gain interpersonal and interprofessional confidence in a complex and
collaborative healthcare context, and the successful transfer of knowledge between
healthcare professionals (Lazarsfeld-Jensen & Bridges, 2012).

It is important to mention, however, that simulation for IPE requires resources, preparation time, and potential financial costs (i.e., equipment costs, staff support); therefore,
the success of a simulation program that will foster the development of IPE competencies is contingent on a program's capacity for sustainability, as well as its ability
to continuously develop and deliver effective simulation-based education at multiple
levels, both to immediate participants and future observers (Lazarsfeld-Jensen & Bridges,
2012). To achieve effective educational results, IPE simulation should ideally be paired
with instructional clinical workshops for the deliberate practice and evaluation of skills,

and close participation with participants to debrief and evaluate leadership skills, communication skills, and teamwork.

Collaboration Tools

The use of technology requires that the technology at hand be easy to use in the learning process. Many of today's students have grown up with technology that is facile to use and provides opportunity for collaboration. Although much has been written about the use of *wikis* for collaboration, Google Docs® has proven to be an easy-to-integrate tool for collaborative learning. Google Docs allows for synchronous and asynchronous viewing and editing, leading to knowledge construction and allowing for more meaningful collaborative learning experiences (Kieser & Golden, 2009). Google Docs can be an invaluable means of maintaining continuity between clinical learning and classroom learning (George, 2012). Google Docs provides students the opportunity to develop interprofessional socialization (IPS) (Khalili, Orchard, Laschinger, & Farah, 2013), regardless of location, and facilitates the inclusion of more students in IPE-related activities. Google Docs allows for "real-time" learning to take place, where faculty can also play an active role either as facilitator or guide.

Social Media

Social media are platforms used by people to create social interactions via the Internet among members of a particular social group. Social media platforms can be text-, video-, picture-, or audio-based, and they allow communication or "social" exchanges to take place synchronously or asynchronously over time. Learning through social media can be both formal and informal, creating a new pedagogical approach to support the current learners of today.

Further understanding generations' use of social medial, as well as delineating generational differences, can be leveraged in fostering IPE. Facebook, Twitter, and Instagram, for example, can connect students to patient-centered care, quality and safety initiatives, and interprofessional collaboration.

Facebook™ is currently the largest social media platform (Pew Research Center, 2014). Facebook allows visual content, pictures, text, and video to be posted to its server by subscribers. Private groups can be created to allow for interactive discussions or content knowledge sharing. Students can follow groups that post content on interprofessional practice, health advocacy, and person-centered care.

Twitter™, a social network platform once favored by younger users, has made its way into health education. The platform enables users to write and read online posts (known as "tweets") that are limited to 140 characters. This free service has more than 500 million active users who generate more than 340 million tweets and 1.6 billion search queries per day (Patient Safety and Quality Council, 2012). It has a diverse group of users, including health professionals, who use Twitter to keep up-to-date. Tweets that are about a particular topic are given a dedicated hashtag (#) (i.e., #simulation, #nursinged) to archive all tweets relating to the specific topic. Hashtags enable users to search for information relating to a topic and check to see what has been added recently.

It is common for delegates from a conference to tweet quotes from speakers or workshops at the conference, and to ascribe an official hashtag designated by the conference organizers; this allows those attending the conference to look at how other delegates are responding to events and has the potential to widen audience participation to beyond those able to physically attend the conference (Gurbani, 2014). Twitter has been keen to leverage IPE as tweets on a particular topic, or hashtags, are submitted by users from varied professions and allow for the open exchange of medical information, ideas, and content asynchronously on its platform.

Blogs

Blogs have become increasingly popular in healthcare and have emerged as a means to quickly disseminate health information across the various professions within the health sciences. Originating from the work *weblog,* a blog is typically a discussion (i.e., conversation thread) through a series of entries, or posts, that are published on the World Wide Web. Primarily textual, a blog can combine text, images, video media, or web links to other resources. Because of the ease with which individuals can access, read, and comment on blog posts, they have quickly become a facile way for learners across all specialties to exchange information.

Contributors to these posts, or *bloggers,* have the opportunity to produce and share their content with interested parties and in the process can build social relations with their readers and fellow bloggers. Therefore, in a sense, blogs can allow learning communities to emerge and/or develop within the health sciences. Because of their quick integration into educational contexts, blogs are commonly used as instructional resources and are now referred to as *edublogs* (i.e., Life in the Fast Lane Medical Blog, the Nursing Site Blog, Academic Life in Emergency Medicine).

Microblogging, the posting of small pieces of content (i.e., text, PDFs, journal article links, images, short videos, or other media) on the web has also become popular. This allows for a more informal and conversational approach to communication, which appeals to those members who wish to make a contribution to the content or dialogue. Examples of microblogging also include Facebook, Twitter, and Instagram.

It is important to note here that content uploaded onto blogs or microblogs is not peer reviewed. Because of the facile nature with which learners can share and exchange information, the validity of content posted on a blog is often not screened or corroborated. Therefore, the content of blogs should always be examined critically, especially in circumstances where recommendations are made for patient care. Professional societies in the health sciences may host and/or sponsor blogs as well; however, the reader of a blog post should verify whether content made immediately available to the public is reviewed or edited in some capacity (i.e., responding to an erroneous post with accurate information).

Apps

An app is short for *application,* which refers to a software program designed for a smartphone or mobile device. New apps are developed every second. Currently, there are more than 300,000 apps available in the Apple™ app store, not to mention those apps that are available in the Google™ Play store. The two key features of using apps in an educational program are to ensure that all students have access to a mobile device and that the app is being used for a meaningful learning experience. When used for student engagement, apps can be an efficient use of students' time, eliminate barriers, and support collaboration. Students can use calendar apps to share schedules and plan accordingly. *Chat apps* allow students the opportunity to engage in knowledge "exchanges" and have direct communication with one another. *Video and photography apps* can help students understand populations/communities and social determinants of health. *Document-sharing apps* can help students develop interprofessional plans of care. Some apps allow students to develop their writing skills. Apps with video features can help students develop patient presentation skills and connect with colleagues in a more personal manner compared to simple text chatting.

Learning Management Systems

Presently, 99 percent of the educational institutions in the United States utilize some form of a learning management system (LMS). Ubiquitous in undergraduate education and beyond, the LMS is the software that provides the learner with an integrated suite of online resources and communication capabilities, either in support of traditional face-to-face courses or fully online courses (Lang & Pirani, 2014). A typical LMS provides its learners with modules (i.e., databases, wikis, and presentation slide decks), facilitates assessments (i.e., tests and/or quizzes), enables instructor/facilitator monitoring of student engagement (i.e., logging on, completing or posting assignments, posting a blog to a discussion thread), and allows for the distribution of grades. For coursework that employs it, the LMS essentially serves as the course's hub for management, communication, and discussion between students and the facilitator, and creation and storage of course-related materials (Lang & Pirani, 2014). Examples of popular LMS programs include BlackBoard, Moodle, Edmodo, and Canvas.

LMS programs and features have also been adapted to nonclassroom and non-academic contexts. In many instances, for example, LMS platforms have been used to organize the products and deliverables produced by work groups, to facilitate dialogue before and after meetings, and to archive projects that have been completed. Given their functionality and forum for the open exchange of information, LMS platforms can play a pivotal role in interprofessional collaboration and education in both academic and nonacademic settings.

Mobile Health

Mobile health (or mHealth) refers to the practice of medicine and public health supported by mobile communication devices (i.e., mobile phones; tablet computers; and personal digital assistants, or PDAs) for health services and health information communication (Adibi, 2015). Mobile communication technologies enable faster communication in remote areas where wireless infrastructure is able to reach more populations. As a result of these technological advances, the capacity for improved access to information and two-way communication has become increasingly available, especially when health-related information is needed most (Agar, 2003).

Mobile health has also emerged as a means of providing larger segments of a population in developing countries access to quality healthcare (Adibi, 2014). Specifically, mHealth-related projects have the potential to provide populations with access to healthcare and health-related information, especially remote populations; improved surveillance of diseases; timely dissemination of public health information and updates; and continuous medical education and training for health providers (Vital Wave Consulting, 2009). As a testament to mHealth's potential, the United Nations (UN) has set initiatives with regard to specific development goals involving mHealth; some of these include "reducing child mortality; improving maternal health; combating HIV and AIDS, malaria, and other diseases; and increasing access to safe drinking water" (United Nations, 2000).

The number of applications within the realm of mHealth is rapidly growing. The UN Foundation and Vodafone Foundation report, as cited in Adibi (2014), presented several application categories within the field, including education and awareness, diagnostic and treatment support, training for healthcare workers, disease and epidemic surveillance, and remote data collection.

A SMART WAY TO INCORPORATE TECHNOLOGY IN INTERPROFESSIONAL PROGRAMS

Clearly stated educational objectives serve as the basis for monitoring an educational program's success in achieving its goals. Sound objectives allow for monitoring the implementation of an educational initiative, assist in setting targets for accountability, and lend to program evaluation (Evaluation Research Team, 2009). SMART objectives (i.e., *specific, measurable, achievable, realistic,* and *timely* objectives) allow the educator to effectively tailor, deliver, and monitor the success of an educational program (Doran, 1981) (Figure 8.3).

Educators interested in applying technological tools to their IPE programming may consider the SMART framework as a means to thoroughly consider the approach to its successful integration. By systematically thinking of the technology at hand within each of these domains, the educator is more likely to choose the technological tool and format best suited to the coursework and its learners.

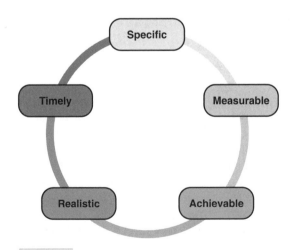

FIGURE 8.3 SMART Objectives.

TABLE 8.1

Using the SMART Approach to Interprofessional Education and Collaborative Practice

SMART Domains	Questions to Ask to Approach IPE Technology Integration
Specific	• What technological tool or application is being used? • Who are the learners? • What value does the particular technological tool have for the overall course? • Will all members of the IPE team benefit from the technology?
Measurable	• How much technology will be integrated into coursework? • Can its impact be captured? • Will its use make a difference in the learning process and how? • Will all members of the IPE team use the technology?
Achievable	• Can the technology being considered be easily used by learners? • Does the technology fit with the goals and objectives of the IPE program? • May its cost or availability pose an obstacle to students across the health professions? • Are certain students from a health profession less likely to use the technology?
Realistic	• Will the technology be easily integrated and paired with course content? • Does the addition of technology enhance the overall value of the educational program? • Will the learners use the technology and appreciate its inclusion into the educational program?
Timely	• Is the technological tool or application best suited for the time course of the educational program? • Over what time frame does the additional technological program need to be completed? • Will the members of the IPE team have time to fully engage in the coursework with extra technological additions?

Through a series of questions, the SMART framework can be applied to the integration of educational programs and/or initiatives. It is meant to serve as a model example for educators to reflect on prior to choosing and applying a technological tool to an interprofessional program. Table 8.1 represents several questions within each domain that educators can ask of the technology being considered. Box 8.1 presents exemplars of the use of technology in IPE and CP learning opportunities.

IMPLICATIONS FOR NURSING EDUCATION

Although this chapter has focused on the student involved in IPE and ways to use technology in IPE, there is a direct impact in the way healthcare consumers use technology. The direct use of technology by patients, their families, communities, and world change the healthcare dynamic significantly. In January 2014, a health survey conducted by the Pew Research Center found that more people than ever have used the Internet— 87 percent of U.S. adults (Pew Research Center, 2014). The survey also found that 72 percent of Internet users looked online for health information, and 70 percent of U.S. adults received information, care, or technology support from a physician or another member of the healthcare team.

BOX 8.1

Eight Exemplars of the Use of Technology in Interprofessional Education and Collaborative Practice Learning Opportunities

The following exemplars offer suggestions as to how educators in the health professions can integrate technology into educational practice across various professions and various learning environments:

- *Social media:* Students following a patient population on Facebook can generate a fair amount of discussion about living with a chronic disease and illustrate how an interprofessional team might be able to manage transitions of care.
- *Root cause analysis:* Structured learning experiences include collective problem solving and group interaction in which clinical practice settings provide an active learning environment for students in interprofessional education (IPE) to transfer knowledge to practice (Wellmon, Gilin, Knauss, & Linn, 2012; Nisbet, Hendry, Rolls, & Field, 2008).
- *Technology-enhanced clinical rounding:* Although a clinical setting is reported to have a positive outcome for practice (Price et al., 2009), several barriers exist that limit students' ability to participate, most notably conflicting clinical rotations schedules. Because Thomas Jefferson University is not immune to this issue, the faculty used technology to enhance the IPE clinical rounding experience by conducting a virtual collaboration for the students who could not physically attend. While utilizing a document tool, students who were clinically based at the patient's bedside collaborated with students who were in other parts of the hospital, and even off-site. Students maintained HIPAA compliance and did not add any identifiable data to the shared document. The nursing student assigned to the patient initiated the document and collaborated with the medical student assigned to the service. The nursing and medical student developed a plan of care and shared it with their colleagues who were off-site for further input. Students utilized the *chat and comment* feature to communicate with each other and handheld and mobile devices for recording and updating document information. An added benefit of this technological initiative was the decrease in physical trips by medical students to the unit for patient updates. In the afternoon, the team was assembled through a video conferencing app on their devices for virtual teaching rounds, and the students delivered a plan of care presentation to the attending physician and the patient.
- *Twitter:* Over the past 5 years, Twitter has revolutionized the exchange of information for health providers practicing emergency medicine. One of the most well-known Twitter medical hashtags is *Free Open Access Medical Education* (abbreviated *#FOAMed*). Since its creation in 2012 by Australian emergency medicine physician Mike Cadogan, it has amassed a following of FOAM enthusiasts across various health disciplines, including pharmacists, nurses, physicians, and emergency medical technicians. The goal of #FOAMed is to share education resources and raise pertinent questions to the emergency medicine community. Twitter posts typically contain medical education content, evidence-based research, best practices, and treatment guidelines (Grundlingh, Harris, & Carley, 2013). FOAM is not exclusive to Twitter, but it uses Twitter as a major forum to link users to emergency medicine resources across the web. Examples of these resources include podcasts, recorded lecture slides, and medical images (i.e., radiographs, electrocardiograms, and ultrasound still images). Resources are posted and shared from health providers across all health professions, further promoting interprofessional collaboration and education in emergency medicine.

In 2012, the Pew Research Center also surveyed Americans on the use of mobile health. Of the U.S. adults surveyed, 52 percent reported using a smartphone for health or medical information. They also found that 19 percent of smartphone users downloaded an app to track and monitor an aspect of their health.

As more and more patients are turning to technology, it is more imperative than ever to have students interact with technology as well. It is also imperative that students start developing the collaborative skills and partnerships currently needed with today's patients.

As noted previously, the Institute of Medicine's *Future of Nursing* report supports practice partnerships with other healthcare professionals; additionally, leadership skills to influence change in health delivery are essential (Institute of Medicine, 2010). Learning together provides opportunities to develop needed skills as a member of a working team. As detailed earlier, the Interprofessional Education Collaborative (IPEC) Expert Panel (2011) report proposed that all healthcare professions students must possess, upon completion of their education, four domains of core competencies to provide integrated, collaborative, high-quality, and cost-effective care. One of the IPEC Core Competencies listed is teamwork. Using technology to bring together teams of healthcare providers, who otherwise would not be able to collaborate on competencies because of logistics, will have a transformative, lifelong effect on quality patient care.

Shifting paradigms in healthcare delivery will require that health professions educators add interprofessional CP to IPE. Healthcare professions students are traditionally socialized to the practice of their respective discipline. Additionally, they must also be socialized to be an active member of the healthcare team. Khalili, Orchard, Laschinger, and Farah (2013) identified the need for IPS and the development of a dual identity for students. This dual identity is the first step toward creating interprofessional CP. IPS has three stages: breaking down barriers, interprofessional role learning, and dual identity development. Students can move toward developing an interprofessional identity by participating in collaborative interprofessional activities using an active learning environment facilitated by technology.

Khalili et al. (2013) state that the stages are not linear but rather are iterative. During the socialization to practice, nursing students develop an identity of their roles and responsibilities in person-centered care, but they also develop leadership skills. While nursing students are developing the knowledge, skills, and attitudes to lead change, they need to be socialized to their role as part of an interprofessional team. While participating in IPE, students, through technology, will develop an innovative skill set that will help them forge new dimensions in healthcare.

CONCLUSION

Technology and its multitude of applications have the potential to transform interprofessional instruction and scholarship by creating new paradigms for collaboration across the health professions. Understanding educational principles for interprofessional pedagogy is of paramount importance in nursing education. Along with the dramatic changes in healthcare, healthcare delivery, and health policy, the role that nurses play has changed from primary caregiver to collaborative partner and promoter. The need to function as an integral partner in patient care has never been louder, and the demand for collaboration with other members from the healthcare team has never been so essential to learning in the health professions.

Although there will be multiple barriers for faculty to overcome to engage in CP, the technological tools discussed in this chapter have the potential to unite teams effectively, and in a timely manner. Applying Bloom's taxonomy, SMART goals, and the TPACK model to the integration of technology in IPE will play a vital role in creating the ideal, patient-centered, team-based approach to high-quality collaborative care.

References

Adibi, S. (2015). *Mobile Health: A Technology Road Map.* New York: Springer.

Adibi, S. (2014). *mHealth Multidisciplinary Verticals.* Boca Raton, FL: CRC Press.

Agar, J. (2003). *Constant Touch: A Global History of the Mobile Phone.* Cambridge, MA: Icon Books Ltd.

American Association of Colleges of Nursing. (2008). *The essentials of baccalaureate education for professional nursing practice.* Washington, DC: Author.

Bloom, B. S., Engelhart, M. D., Furst, E. J., Hill, W. H., & Krathwohl, D. R. (1956). *Taxonomy of educational objectives, Handbook I: The cognitive domain.* New York: David McKay.

Coomes, M. D., & DeBard, R. (Eds.). (2004). *Serving the millennial generation.* San Francisco. Jossey-Bass.

Decker, S., Sportsman, S., Puetz, L., & Ballinger, L. (2008). The evolution of simulation and its contribution to competency. *Journal of Continuing Education in Nursing, 39*(2), 74–80.

Doran, G. T. (1981). There's a S.M.A.R.T way to write management's goals and objectives. *Management Review, 70*(11), 35–36.

EdTechReview. (2013). Steps for improving learning outcomes with technology. Retrieved June 7, 2016, from http:// edtechreview.in/trends-insights/ insights/864-steps-for-improving-learning- outcomes-with-technology

Evaluation Research Team, Department of Health and Human Services, Centers for Disease Control and Prevention. (2009). Writing SMART objectives. *Evaluation Briefs* (No. 3b). Retrieved June 7, 2016, from https://www.cdc.gov/healthyyouth/ evaluation/pdf/brief3b.pdf

George, D. R. (2012). Using Google Docs to enhance medical student reflection. *Medical Education, 46,* 504–505. doi:10.1111/j. 1365-2923.2012.04233.x

Graesser, A. C., Chipman, P., & King, B. (2008). Computer-mediated technologies. In J. M. Spector, M. D. Merrill, J. Van Merrienboer, & M. Driscoll (Eds.), *Handbook of research for educational communications and tech- nology* (3rd ed., pp. 211–224). New York: Routledge.

Grundlingh, J., Harris, T., & Carley, S. (2013). FOAM: The Internet, social media and medi- cal education. *Emergency Medicine Journal,* 2013(Suppl.), 2–4.

Gurbani, C. (2014). How can Twitter support your studies? *Student BMJ.* Retrieved June 7, 2016, from http://www.medscape.com/ viewarticle/829363_1

Ho, K., Jarvis-Selinger, S., Norman, C., Li, L., Olatunbosun, T., Cressman, C., et al. (2010). Electronic communities of practice: Guide- lines from a project. *Journal of Continuing Education in the Health Professions, 30*(2), 139–143.

Institute of Medicine. (2010). *The future of nursing: Leading change, advancing health.* Washington, DC: National Academies Press.

Interprofessional Education Collaborative Expert Panel. (2011). *Core competencies for interprofessional collaborative practice: Report of an expert panel.* Washington, DC: Interprofessional Education Collaborative.

Interprofessional Education and Healthcare Simulation Symposium. (2012). Society for Simulation in Healthcare, the Josiah Macy

Jr. Foundation, and the National League for Nursing.

Khalili, H., Orchard, C., Laschinger, H. K. S., & Farah, R. (2013). An interprofessional socialization framework for developing an interprofessional identity among health professions students. *Journal of Interprofessional Care, 27*(6), 448–453.

Kieser, A. L., & Golden, F. O. (2009). Using online office applications. *Distance Learning, 6*(1), 41–46.

Lang, L., & Pirani, J. A. (2014). The learning management system evolution: CDS Spotlight Report. *Educause Center for Analysis and Research.* Retrieved June 7, 2016, from https://net.educause.edu/ir/library/pdf/ERB1405.pdf

Lazarsfeld-Jensen, A., & Bridges, D. (2012). Simulation as a vehicle for interprofessional education. Proceedings of the Practice Education and Training (GPET) Conference, Australia.

Koehler, M. J., & Mishra, P. (2008). Introducing TPCK. In AACTE Committee on Innovation and Technology (Ed.), *The handbook of technological pedagogical content knowledge (TPCK) for educators* (pp. 3–29). New York: American Association of Colleges of Teacher Education.

Nisbet, G., Hendry, G. D., Rolls, G., & Field, M. J. (2008). Interprofessional learning for pre-qualification healthcare students: An outcomes-based evaluation. *Journal of Interprofessional Care, 22*(1), 57–68.

Oandasan, I., & Reeves, S. (2005). Key elements for interprofessional education. Part 1: The learner, the educator, and the learning context. *Journal of Interprofessional Care, 19*, 21–38.

Patient Safety and Quality Council. (2012). *Twitter for health care professionals.* Retrieved June 7, 2016, from https://www.dur.ac.uk/resources/public.health/leading-transformation/event2/Twitter-For-Health-Care-Professionals.pdf

Pew Research Center. (2014). *Social media update 2014.* Retrieved June 7, 2016, from http://www.pewinternet.org/2015/01/09/social-media-update-2014/

Pew Research Center. (2015). *Health fact sheet.* Retrieved June 7, 2016, from http://www.pewinternet.org/fact-sheets/health-fact-sheet/

Price, D., Howard, M., Hilts, L., Dolovich, L., McCarthy, L., Walsh, A. E., et al. (2009). Interprofessional education in academic family medicine teaching units: A functional program and culture. *Canadian Family Physician, 55*(9), 901–901.

Shaffer, K. (2014). *Enhancing interprofessional education with technology.* Doctoral Dissertation, University of Delaware. Available at http://search.proquest.com/docview/1661456521

Speakman, E. (2015). *A vision for interprofessional collaboration in education and practice, a living document from the national league for nursing.* National League for Nursing.

Thibault, G. E. (2013). Reforming health professions education will require culture change and closer ties between classroom and practice. *Health Affairs, 32*(11), 1928–1932.

United Nations. (2000). *United Nations millennium declaration.* General Assembly Resolution 55/2. New York: Author.

Vital Wave Consulting. (2009). *mHealth for Development: The opportunity of mobile technology for healthcare in the developing world.* Washington, DC: United Nations Foundation.

Wellmon, R., Gilin, B., Knauss, L., & Linn, M. I. (2012). Changes in student attitudes toward interprofessional learning and collaboration arising from a case-based educational experience. *Journal of Allied Health, 41*(1), 26–34.

Wenger, E. (1998). *Communities of practice: Learning, meaning, and identity* (6th ed.). Cambridge, MA: Cambridge University Press.

West Midland Family Center (WMFC). Generational Differences Chart Traditionalists Baby Boomers Generation X Millennials Birth Years 1900–1945 1946–1964 1965–1980 (1977–1994). Retrieved July, 7, 2016, from http://www.wmfc.org/uploads/GenerationalDifferencesChart.pdf

9

Interprofessional Education and Simulation: Building a Culture of Communication and Teamwork for Patient Safety

John J. Duffy, DNP, MSN, RN, CCRN
Alan T. Forstater, MD, FACEP
Anne Marie Pettit, MSN, RN

Good communication skills and effective teamwork are the core components that give patient care and patient safety top priority to achieve positive outcomes. Interprofessional education (IPE) is an educational strategy used to train healthcare professionals and future healthcare professionals to enhance teamwork and improve communication and quality of care (Carlson, 2011). Nursing and nursing education has particularly been interested in preparing nurses with the knowledge, skills, and attitudes (KSAs) necessary to continuously improve the quality and safety of healthcare (www.qsen.org).

PATIENT SAFETY

Patient safety moved to the forefront of healthcare with the release in 1999 of the Institute of Medicine (IOM) landmark report, *To Err Is Human: Building a Safer Health System.* This IOM report estimated that up to one million people were injured and "98,000 died annually in the United States as a result of medical errors" (Kohn, Corrigan, & Donaldson, 1999, p. 11).

In the *To Err Is Human* report, the IOM defined *error* as "the failure of a planned action to be completed as intended (i.e., error of execution) or the use of a wrong plan to achieve an aim (i.e., error of planning)," an *adverse event* as "an injury caused by medical management rather than the underlying condition of the patient," and a *preventable adverse event* as an adverse event attributable to error (Kohn et al., 1999, p. 21). The report began by observing that "errors can be prevented by designing systems that make it hard for people to do the wrong thing and easy for people to do the right thing" (Ulrich & Kear, 2014, p. 448). Interestingly, the nature of medical errors has demonstrated that most often the root causes of the error are embedded in the system itself.

In 2001, the IOM published *Crossing the Quality Chasm: A New Health System for the 21st Century,* further detailing the changes needed to ensure patient safety as well as looking at other quality issues. Teamwork is cited as essential in caring for patients with complex problems. The authors strongly suggest "placing more stress on teaching evidence-based practice and providing more opportunities for interdisciplinary training" (Institute of Medicine [IOM], 2001, p. 6).

An example of communication failure is the Sue Sheridan case. Sue became involved in patient safety after her family experienced two serious medical system failures. Their son, Cal, suffered brain damage called *kernicterus* 5 days after birth in 1995 when the family's concerns were ignored and his neonatal jaundice was left untreated. Her husband, Pat, died in 2002 after his pathology report of spinal cancer failed to be communicated accurately to his surgeon during his original operation. In 2003, Sue cofounded Consumers Advancing Patient Safety (www.patientsafety.org), a nonprofit organization that seeks a safe, compassionate, and just healthcare system through proactive partnership between consumers and providers of care. In 2004, Sue was asked to lead the World Health Organization's Patients for Patient Safety Initiative (http://www.who.int/patientsafety/information_centre/interviews/sheridan/en).

In 2004, the Institute for Healthcare Improvement launched the 100,000 Lives Campaign with the slogan, "Some is not a number—Soon is not a time," to improve patient care and reduce morbidity and mortality in American healthcare. The campaign focus is on six key interventions: rapid response teams, improved care for acute myocardial infarction, prevention of adverse drug events, prevention of central line-associated bloodstream infections, prevention of surgical site infections, and prevention of ventilator-associated pneumonia (Institute for Healthcare Improvement, 2004).

In 2002, the Joint Commission on the Accreditation of Healthcare Organizations (JAHCO) established National Patient Safety Goals (NPSGs) to improve patient safety by assisting healthcare organizations to address specific areas of concern with regard to patient safety. On January 1, 2003, the first NPSGs highlighted areas of concern for all healthcare institutions. All were related to teamwork and communication.

Implementation of these standards would ensure that all patients would experience the safest, highest-quality, best-value healthcare across all settings, creating a culture change in healthcare delivery. In 2008, the Joint Commission noted that "safety and quality of patient care is dependent on teamwork, communication and a collaborative work environment" (Joint Commission, 2008, p. 1). Understanding and optimizing team performance and collaboration among team members is a core responsibility of all healthcare team members.

INTERPROFESSIONAL EDUCATION AND PATIENT SAFETY

As noted previously, *interprofessional education* is defined as "when students from two or more professions learn about, from and with each other to enable effective collaboration and improve health outcomes" (World Health Organization, 2010, p. 10). IPE can be used to build a culture of communication and teamwork from the beginning training of all healthcare professionals. As described earlier, the Interprofessional Education Collaborative (IPEC) Expert Panel (2011) report presented an expectation of effective interprofessional collaborative practice (CP), beginning with the development of interprofessional competencies for health profession students who actively work as members of clinical teams as part of their learning process (Interprofessional Education Collaborative [IPEC] Expert Panel, 2011). When newly graduated health professionals enter the workforce, they should be competent in the essential skills of teamwork and team-based care, which would improve patient safety outcomes in the area of healthcare in which they are employed. The development of interprofessional collaborative competencies through IPE requires moving beyond discipline-specific educational efforts toward engaging students of different professions in interactive learning with each other. Being able to work effectively as members of clinical teams while in the student role is a fundamental part of that learning. The existing educational system is not preparing health professionals for teamwork (Wilhaus et al., 2012). The four IPEC Core Competency domains of values/ethics for interprofessional practice, roles/responsibilities, interprofessional communication, and teams/teamwork (IPEC Expert Panel, 2011) remain an essential framework to build a culture of patient safety.

As described in Chapter 8, the Society for Simulation in Healthcare (SSH) and the National League for Nursing (NLN) met to discuss and identify an opportunity to enhance IPE outcomes by better understanding and leveraging the intersection between IPE and simulation (NLN, 2011). The SSH believes that simulation is an effective vehicle for achieving and evaluating the interprofessional competencies. The American Association of Colleges of Nursing (AACN) led a national effort designed to enhance the ability of nurse faculty to effectively develop quality and safety competencies among graduates of their programs. The AACN hosted a series of regional Quality and Safety Education for Nurses (QSEN) Faculty Development Institutes. The program gave nurse faculty key training and information to improve their curricula. The framework was based on recommendations from the IOM (2003) to prepare all health professionals with six core competencies—patient-centered care, teamwork and collaboration, evidence-based care, quality improvement, safety, and informatics, providing the KSAs essential to achieve each competency. The goal of the safety competency is to "minimize risk of harm to patients and providers through both system effectiveness and individual performance" (Cronenwett et al., 2007, p. 128).

TEAMWORK AND COMMUNICATION

Examples of team training and simulation in healthcare are relatively sparse (Aron & Headrick, 2002, p. 170). "Even though the delivery of care requires teamwork, members of these teams are rarely trained together; they often come from separate disciplines and diverse educational programs" (King et al., 2008, p. 5). Often the students are on the same campus but are not aware of what the other health professions are being taught. When healthcare professionals are not communicating effectively, patient safety is at risk for several reasons: lack of critical information, misinterpretation of information, unclear orders over the telephone, and overlooked changes in status (O'Daniel & Rosenstein, 2008). Lack of communication creates situations where medical errors can occur. These errors have the potential to cause severe injury or unexpected patient death.

"Unfortunately, many health care workers are used to poor communication and teamwork, as a result of a culture of low expectations that has developed in many health care settings" (O'Daniel & Rosenstein, 2008, p. 2-273). "Teaching people how to speak up and create the dynamic where they will express their concerns is a key factor in safety" (Leonard, Graham, & Bonacum, p. i86). Effective communication can lead to the following positive outcomes: improved information flow, more effective interventions, improved safety, enhanced employee morale, increased patient and family satisfaction, and decreased lengths of stay. Therefore, implementing systems to facilitate team communication can substantially improve quality.

Communication problems have been shown to be responsible for medical errors 70 percent of the time (Studdert, Brennan, & Thomas, 2002). These communication errors may be errors of commission—that is, something was stated incorrectly or misunderstood. Alternatively, they may be communication errors of omission—that is, by not speaking up when a problem or concern is suspected or simply leaving key information out of the communication. The traditional hierarchy, placing the physician at the top, can be intimidating to the nurse, who is afraid that he or she may be perceived as questioning the doctor and the doctor may feel that his or her authority is being usurped when questioned. Alternatively, nonphysicians may hesitate to question the doctor, deferring to his or her knowledge or experience simply because of position in the hierarchy, despite the fact that the nurse or other professional may have valuable and valid information about the patient's condition. This has been referred to as the halo effect, depicting the proverbial halo adorning a physician or anyone higher in the hierarchy (Agency for Healthcare Research and Quality [AHRQ], 2014).

This aura attributed to anyone may prevent someone from speaking up and can lead to a preventable medical error. There are multiple reasons someone with a patient safety concern may hesitate to speak up, including fear of embarrassment if he or she were wrong and fear of retribution for challenging someone in authority. If the physician or someone in authority has a history of acting in an intimidating manner, that would make the individual seem to be unapproachable (Sutcliffe, Lewton, & Rosenthal, 2004). One solution is to train all individuals to expect interprofessional communication that furthermore is structured in a way that requires gathering and transmitting of essential information in an organized fashion. Effective teams need assurance that questioning a colleague is not only acceptable but is encouraged, expected, and appreciated. Furthermore, speaking up about a safety concern should be viewed as supportive, to help a colleague avoid an error, rather than an attempt to question that colleague's knowledge or authority. We must remind our students and colleagues that our top priority is our patients' care and safety.

"The complexity of medical care, coupled with the inherent limitations of human performance, make it critically important that clinicians have standardized communication tools, create an environment in which individuals can speak up and express concerns, and share common 'critical language' to alert team members to unsafe situations" (O'Daniel & Rosenstein, 2008, p. 4,5). Other fields that deal with or impact public safety, such as firefighters, the airline industry, and the nuclear energy industry, work in teams that rely heavily on accurate concise information exchange and must react quickly to changing situations. Research shows that in these fields, personnel have had success in training together using standardized proven methods of communication, improving teamwork, and minimizing risk (O'Daniel & Rosenstein, 2008). A systematic review done by Weaver et al. (2013) "revealed that 16 of the 20 studies they examined reported statistically significant improvement in staff perceptions of safety culture (after an intervention to improve team skills or communication). In addition, five reported improvements in care processes (for example, decreased care delays or increased use of structured communication) and seven reported improvements in patient safety outcomes (for example, errors resulting in harm or reductions in adverse outcomes index" (p. 371).

TEAM-BASED APPROACH

Multiple patient safety organizations have recommended that healthcare organizations develop a team-based approach and train their teams accordingly to prevent medical errors in response to the IOM report on the crisis in patient safety, which stated that at least 98,000 lives were lost to medical error annually (Kohn et al., 1999). In 2010, the National Quality Forum called for a "proactive systematic organization-wide approach to developing team-based care through teamwork training, skill building and team-led performance improvement interventions that reduce preventable patient harm" (Meyer, Denham, & Battles, 2010, p. 8). Sutcliffe, Lewton, and Rosenthal (2004) highlighted the role of poor communication among team members in medical errors and emphasized the importance of improving staff communication to prevent errors. The Committee on Quality of Health Care in America recommended the development of multidisciplinary team training programs based on proven methods such as crew resource management (CRM) (IOM, 2001).

CREW RESOURCE MANAGEMENT

United Airlines spearheaded the earliest version of CRM in the airline industry after a series of airline disasters in the 1970s. Despite initial doubts by some, the results were so positive that skeptics were swayed and the concept was embraced by all airlines. Since then, the National Aeronautics and Space Administration (NASA) and myriad psychologists, sociologists, and managerial experts contributed to studies that molded CRM into its current form. Orasanu and Fischer (2008) emphasize that some features of effective communication on the airline flight deck could be applicable to the healthcare environment. They include building a shared mental model, establishing a positive climate through briefings, monitoring to prevent problems and errors, using explicit and effective language, and standardizing and procedural communication.

An essential component of CRM training is simulation, which provides an opportunity for teams to problem solve challenging situations by utilizing their best team communication skills and team behaviors. In response to the challenge by the IOM to develop a program modeled after CRM to address the patient safety problem, the Department of Defense (DoD) and the Agency for Healthcare Research and Quality (AHRQ) used some of the same principles of CRM to develop TeamSTEPPS®, an acronym for Team Strategies and Tools to Enhance Performance and Patient Safety.

TeamSTEPPS®

TeamSTEPPS® is a program "based on twenty-five years of research on teamwork, team training and culture change" (King et al., 2008, p. 5) and draws on the DoD's expertise in medical and nonmedical team training and performance, as well as the extensive research in patient safety and healthcare quality (Clancy & Tornberg, 2007). Released in the public domain in November 2006, TeamSTEPPS® training is intended to clarify team roles and responsibilities and optimize the use of information, people, and resources to achieve the best clinical outcomes for patients (AHRQ, 2015). By providing tools and strategies to cultivate the core teamwork competencies of leadership, situation monitoring, mutual support, and communication, TeamSTEPPS® aims to increase team awareness through a shared mental model (Ferguson, 2008). "Based on the concept of 'just culture,' the program seeks to foster an environment of mutual respect wherein all members of the team feel comfortable voicing patient safety concerns irrespective of their perceived positions or roles" (Clancy & Tornberg, 2007, p. 216). "TeamSTEPPS® aims to transform the culture of an organization by establishing a common language for talking about communication and teamwork failures; by bridging professional divides and leveling hierarchy; by providing teachable-learnable skills and actions to practice; and by conceptualizing the patient as a valued team member" (Coburn & Gage-Croll, 2011, p. 3).

To make the program available to as many people and institutions as possible, the AHRQ has made training materials available via the website and has sanctioned and sponsored training sites with courses around the country to train master trainers who can then return to their home institutions to train colleagues there and infuse TeamSTEPPS® principles in the development of patient safety and performance improvement programs. Simulation is an ideal vehicle to train professionals with the skills they will need to successfully and safely treat patients. Team training, and specifically TeamSTEPPS® training, is best experienced and reinforced with simulation where professionals in a safe environment experience scenarios that allow them to practice team behaviors learned in the program.

INTERPROFESSIONAL EDUCATION AND HEALTHCARE SIMULATION

At the 2012 Invitational Meeting of Key Stakeholders in Interprofessional Education and Healthcare Simulation, the consensus of this interprofessional group of 29 revealed "that the climate is indeed ripe to advance safety and improve quality care through simulation-enhanced IPE" (Wilhaus et al., 2012, p. 19). Effective teamwork requires specific education directed at educating healthcare providers to be effective team members. Health professions education currently offers limited opportunities for practiced interaction with students of other disciplines. Simulation offers an opportunity to address these needs. The current climate for IPE is often poorly defined, inconsistent, fragmented, and nonstandardized. Common concerns expressed include the traditional compartmentalization of disciplines and regulatory bodies. IPE in general and simulation-enhanced IPE efforts in particular vary across the organizations in terms of scope, integration, purpose, and longevity. Role confusion within each profession was seen as a hindrance to implementing simulation-enhanced IPE, as was the cost for purchasing equipment, space in existing simulation centers, and the time necessary for planning and implementation. Initial reports "reveal that students who participated in team training scored higher on team based/IPE competencies" (Wilhaus et al., 2012, p. 17).

With a goal of improving patient safety and the quality of healthcare, IPE can help to develop effective interprofessional practice. Simulation is an excellent active learning method to train healthcare providers, not only about knowledge within their discipline but also in interprofessional learning (Wilhaus et al., 2012). "Discussion and collaboration among health disciplines, professional organizations, safety advocates, and other healthcare leaders around the use of simulation are effective ways to initiate and stimulate IPE endeavors" (Wilhaus et al., 2012, p. 19).

SIMULATION AND INTERPROFESSIONAL EDUCATION

Nursing educators throughout the country have discussed the use of simulation as an accepted substitute for at least a portion of the student's clinical experiences. Benner, Sutphen, Leonard, and Day (2010) recommended the use of simulation as an essential component in the radical transformation of nursing education. These authors recommend that the National Council of State Boards of Nursing (NCSBN) develop three national simulation examinations of performance. The first performance assessment should occur at the beginning of the last year of nursing school. The second test should be given at the same time as, and in conjunction with, the present National Council Licensure Examination (NCLEX-RN©). The final proposed test would be given at the end of a 1-year postlicensure residency. These examinations would be given in simulation laboratories using standardized patient actors (Benner et al., 2010).

The NCSBN predicts that simulation will increasingly be used as an alternative to clinical experiences (National Council of State Boards of Nursing, 2005). Although simulation will never completely replace hospital clinical rotations, many states are considering permitting a percentage of simulation to count as clinical time. In 2014, the NCSBN concluded a multistate study, the *Longitudinal, Randomized, Controlled Study Replacing Clinical Hours With Simulation in Prelicensure Nursing Education,* which examined the use of simulation in prelicensure nursing education (Hayden, Smiley, Alexander, Kardong-Edgren, & Jeffries, 2014). This study substituted high-quality simulation experiences for up to half of traditional clinical hours, measuring comparable end-of-program educational outcomes. The key component of this study is that each of the 10 participating nursing programs were randomly assigned to one of three groups that substituted simulation for traditional clinical experience by 10 percent, 25 percent, and 50 percent. The study began in the fall semester of 2011 with the first clinical nursing course and continued throughout the core clinical courses to graduation in May 2013. Students were assessed on clinical competency and nursing knowledge. The study rated how well students perceived that their learning needs were met in both the clinical and simulation environments. A sample of 666 students completed the study requirements at the time of graduation. This study "provides substantial evidence that up to 50% simulation can be effectively substituted for traditional clinical experience in all prelicensure core nursing courses under conditions comparable to those described in the study. These conditions include faculty members who are formally trained in simulation pedagogy, an adequate number of faculty members to support the student learners, subject matter experts who conduct theory-based debriefing, and equipment and supplies to create a realistic environment" (Hayden et al., 2014, p. s38). This research found that there were no meaningful differences between the groups in critical thinking, clinical competency, and overall readiness for practice as rated by managers at 6 weeks, 3 months and 6 months after working in a clinical position (Hayden et al., 2014).

High-fidelity simulation (HFS) is a learner-centered form of experiential learning that integrates the cognitive, psychomotor, and affective domains of learning (Nickerson, Morrison, & Pollard, 2011). Clinical challenges are created by an experienced faculty simulationist who employs highly sophisticated computerized manikins or standardized patients to create an authentic clinical scenario. HFS can be used to provide interprofessional, patient-centered clinical experiences that challenge students in the health professions with rare, high-acuity, interprofessional clinical scenarios. Ongoing innovations in technology allow simulation centers the ability to replicate a realistic patient encounter that clinically challenges a team of learners.

Unlike traditional clinical rotations, instruction in a simulation center can be standardized to meet program objectives. Transference of skills learned in the simulation center may prepare the learners to face interprofessional clinical situations in their future practice environment. Fisher and King (2013) found that simulation exposes students to a broad range of experiences while in a safe environment and that the learned skills transfer to the practitioner's clinical practice. Simulations allow learners to repeatedly practice requisite skills without risking harm to any patients. The use of simulation as a teaching andragogy challenges the interprofessional learner in a safe, simulated learning environment that affords the learners an opportunity to perform clinical skills, to test critical decision-making abilities related to patient care management, and the chance to function as members of an interprofessional team (Jeffries, 2005). Gaba (2004) defines *simulation* as a "technique, not a technology, to replace or amplify real experiences with guided experiences, often immersive in nature, that evoke or replicate substantial aspects of the real world in a fully interactive fashion. 'Immersive' conveys the sense that participants have of being immersed in a task or setting as they would if it were the real world" (p. i2).

EFFECTIVE INTERPROFESSIONAL EDUCATION SIMULATION

A prevalent challenge in IPE simulation efforts are prebriefing student leveling and writing thoughtful IPE clinical scenarios that include components appropriate for all respective professions that will be participating in the simulation. The scenario will not work if the objectives fail to engage one group or intimidate another. All participants from the various disciplines need to be on a level playing field. For example, a second-year medical student and a fourth-semester nursing student in a clinical scenario are largely mismatched because of how the students are exposed to their clinical education at varying times within their individual curricula. Attempting to retrofit an HFS scenario to level of experience is a challenge and remains foremost in the minds of the scenarios authors. The facilitator must always be aware of potential vulnerability of the learners who have diverse clinical experience and create a safe, supportive, and nonthreatening learning environment. Developing a climate of respect, mutual trust, and acceptance is imperative.

A traditional prebriefing stage of the simulation is where learners receive physical, hands-on orientation to the simulation. During prebriefing, the learners are given the rules of engagement and are asked to commit to a learning contract that will include their agreement to be polite, respectful, and curious. The learner should be asked to commit to exhibiting professional behavior, respecting a professional learning environment, suspending disbelief, accepting a fictional contract, adhering to a contract of strict confidentiality, and agreeing to be active participants in critical reflection during debriefing. Creating this type of environment is essential to support the learner's self-reflective evaluation during debriefing. The prebriefing activities help to set the stage for the scenario, assisting participants in outlining scenario objectives and communicating the patient presentation, roles, tasks, time allotment, and orientation to equipment and the general environment (Meakim et al., 2013).

Immediate postscenario debriefing affords opportunities for both self- and peer reflection that enhances student-centered learning. The goals of debriefing are for participants to clarify, analyze, and synthesize information and reactions to the simulation to improve their future performance in similar situations (Rudolph, Simon, Rivard, Dufresne, & Raemer, 2007). *Debriefing* is defined as a facilitator-led participant discussion on real or simulated events, reflection, and assimilation of activities into the learner's cognition to produce long-lasting learning (Fanning & Gaba, 2007). Jeffries (2005) states that "debriefing activity reinforces the positive aspects of the experience and encourages reflective learning, which allows the participant to link theory to practice and research, think critically, and discuss how to intervene professionally in very complex situations" (p. 101). An effective approach to debriefing is the method of debriefing with good judgment. This method presumes that the learner's actions are an inevitable result of their "frames," which are comprised of such things as knowledge, assumptions, and feelings that drive their actions. The debriefer's job is that of a "cognitive detective," who tries to discover, through genuine curiosity and inquiry, what those frames are and how they influenced the learner's action in the simulation. This approach includes a conversational technique designed to bring the judgment of the debriefer and the frames of the learner to light. The technique pairs advocacy and inquiry. "Advocacy is a type of speech that includes an objective observation about and subjective judgment of the trainees' actions. Inquiry is a genuinely curious question that attempts to illuminate the trainee's frame in relation to the action described in the instructor's advocacy" (Rudolph, Simon, Dufresne, & Raemer, 2006, p. 49).

UTILIZING TeamSTEPPS®: AN EXEMPLAR

At Thomas Jefferson University, the Jefferson Center for Interprofessional Education (JCIPE) has supported multiple workshops throughout the institution using TeamSTEPPS® principles. Each workshop has been designed to meet the needs of the experience level and needs of the audience whether they are first-year students or experienced clinicians. The workshops are all interprofessional, range from 2 to 4 hours, and usually proceed in the following format: a brief didactic introduction with video clips to demonstrate the core concepts; a simulation-based experience involving the learner as either a participant or an engaged observer; and other interactive components, such as team-building exercises and issue-based brainstorming sessions. Each workshop is uniquely designed for the audience.

TeamSTEPPS® Workshops for Students at Thomas Jefferson University

The first TeamSTEPPS® workshop was held as a pilot for a volunteer group of senior students from various schools: medical, nursing, physical and occupational therapy, radiologic sciences, and couple and family therapy. After a brief introduction to TeamSTEPPS® skills, some video clips available on the AHRQ website, and a team-building exercise, the students were challenged with two simulation cases to apply their knowledge and practice their team-based skills. One case was a cerebrovascular accident patient who fell and seized while in the rehabilitation gym. This scenario required attention to the cervical spine to avoid further injury and attention to the brain to rule out subdural hematoma. It also involved a member of the simulation team acting as a confederate portraying a family member. This scenario challenged the team to rely on their problem-solving skills, as well as team skills, to find the best solution to the problems. In addition to practicing teamwork skills with emphasis on "speaking up," students learned the role of each profession in managing the case and gained an appreciation for the skill set of each other's health profession. The second simulation scenario involved a patient who had a cardiac arrest in the magnetic resonance imaging (MRI) suite. This case focused on the TeamSTEPPS® principle of situational awareness, dealing with the restrictions to access in the MRI suite and the high-stakes interaction of team members in a cardiac resuscitation. Debriefing provided the students an opportunity to reflect on their interaction with other team members' values and abilities, as well as their use of teamwork skills (Forstater, Speakman, Pettit, & Duffy, 2015).

Another student workshop included the Health Mentors Program, an IPE program for entry-level students at Thomas Jefferson University that forms interprofessional teams who interact with a patient in the community who is dealing with a chronic health issue. This simulation scenario involved teams of interprofessional students in a shopping mall offering free health screening, who are suddenly tasked with giving medical support after a catastrophic event. Students tended to people with minor illnesses or injuries and practiced using TeamSTEPPS® to facilitate teamwork and communication.

Regardless of the topic or audience, all workshops were interprofessional and engaged the learner in active learning experiences maximized by facilitated debriefings. During the debriefing sessions, students, with the help of experienced facilitators, had an opportunity to reflect on their team skills, how well the team managed the patients' care, and how well they interacted as team members. It is important to note that although the medical aspects of the cases are discussed, the emphasis of the debriefing was on the team interaction. Evaluations of the various workshops have consistently shown that the majority of participants learned the knowledge content, thought that the workshops' objectives were met, and valued the opportunity to experience an interprofessional clinical simulation. In addition, participants noted that the debriefing allowed them to focus on mastering effective teamwork rather than only solving the healthcare issue.

TeamSTEPPS® Workshops for Staff at Thomas Jefferson University

A TeamSTEPPS® course for faculty, clinicians, and staff was created and offered throughout the Jefferson system. This highly interactive unique TeamSTEPPS® course was designed using simulation, role-playing, and didactic strategies that emphasized collaborative and active learning. The challenge was to bring professionals from all clinical and academic departments with various clinical and nonclinical roles and responsibilities together and to train them to work together effectively and safely in teams.

As a result of the system-wide TeamSTEPPS® program, a course was developed specifically for a clinical department using the Primary Care Version of TeamSTEPPS®. This course utilized the tenets of TeamSTEPPS® but added simulation scenarios that were outpatient focused, enabling the participants who worked in the primary care setting the ability to relate more easily to the training.

NURSING IMPLICATIONS

For nursing, the healthcare delivery system continues to change dramatically. Kirsh and Boysen (2010) noted that achieving greater patient safety requires a fundamental culture change across all phases of medical education. They describe five factors that are critical to success: explicit leadership from the top, early engagement of students in the health professions, having residents teach others about patient safety, the use of information technology, and promoting teamwork among health professions. This is also true of nursing education. As noted previously, the use of simulation is an appropriate and sanctioned (NCSBN) skills' acquisition technique in nursing education. Concomitantly, using interprofessional simulation training experiences with students from multiple professions teaches team-based skills.

Team training and simulation are labor and time intensive, and they require a commitment of significant resources, especially when designed with facilitated small group interaction and simulation with debriefing. To create a culture of safety, students must be allowed to practice together, learn how to engage with one another, and understand how each of their respective professions approaches care delivery. Nurse educators, regardless of the program plan of study, need to find meaningful team-based learning opportunities to prepare their students to become effective members and leaders in healthcare delivery systems that promote and sustain a culture of patient safety. As mentioned earlier, to implement a change in healthcare delivery that impacts patient safety, there must be buy-in from all involved. "Team training can result in transformational change in safety culture when the work environment supports transfer of learning to behavior" (Jones, Skinner, High, & Reiter-Palmon, 2013, pp. 402–403). As the work environment moves toward team-based care, it behooves nurse educators to provide opportunities that prepare students to function as vital members of the healthcare team.

CONCLUSION

Patient safety is not an option but a mandate. Good communication skills and effective teamwork are essential to patient safety and positive outcomes. Patient safety experts have emphasized the importance of IPE as a strategy to train healthcare professionals to improve communication and teamwork, and thus the quality of care. IPE with a focus on patient safety is consistent with QSEN principles. Simulation is an ideal way to teach these principles while maximizing learning and minimizing risk during the learning experience. The acceptance of simulation as an alternative in nursing education to live clinical experience paves the way for increased opportunity to use simulation to teach teamwork skills. Learning takes place as students or professionals practice these skills and is enhanced and reinforced when an experienced facilitator debriefs the learners, giving them the time to reflect on team values and their own ability to function well in interprofessional teams. TeamSTEPPS® is one widely accepted training program that can be used to standardize communication and improve teamwork skills with a goal toward patient safety. By teaching team skills to nursing students or staff in an IPE format with simulation, they have the opportunity to practice these new skills and demonstrate that they can incorporate them into their nursing practice.

References

Agency for Healthcare Research and Quality. (2014). Glossary. Retrieved June 7, 2016, from http://www.ahrq.gov/professionals/education/curriculum-tools/teamstepps/longtermcare/references/glossary.html

Aron, D., & Headrick, L. (2002). Educating physicians prepared to improve care and safety is no accident: It requires a systematic approach. *Quality and Safety in Health Care, 11*(2), 168–173.

Benner, P., Sutphen, M., Leonard, V., & Day, L. (2010). *Educating nurses: A call for radical transformation*. San Francisco, CA: Jossey-Bass.

Carlson, E., Pilhammar, E., & Wann-Hansson, C. (2011). The team builder: The role of nurses facilitating interprofessional student teams at a Swedish clinical training ward. *Nurse Education in Practice, 11*(5), 309–313.

Clancy, C., & Tornberg, D. (2007). TeamSTEPPS: Assuring optimal teamwork in clinical settings. *American Journal of Medical Quality, 22*(3), 214–217.

Coburn, A., & Gage-Croll, Z. (2011). Improving hospital patient safety through teamwork: The use of TeamSTEPPS in critical access hospitals. *Challenge, 5*(7), 1–12.

Cronenwett, L., Sherwood, G., Barnsteiner, J., Disch, J., Johnson, J., Mitchell, P., et al. (2007). Quality and safety education for nurses. *Nursing Outlook, 55*(3), 122–131.

Fanning, R., & Gaba, D. (2007). The role of debriefing in simulation-based learning. *Simulation in Healthcare, 2*(2), 115–125.

Ferguson, S. (2008). TeamSTEPPS: Integrating teamwork principles into adult health/medical-surgical practice. *Medsurg Nursing, 17*(2), 122–125.

Fisher, D., & King, L. (2013). An integrative literature review on preparing nursing students through simulation to recognize and respond to the deteriorating patient. *Journal of Advanced Nursing, 69*(11), 2375–2388. doi:10.1111/jan.12174

Forstater, A., Speakman, E., Petit, A., & Duffy, J. (2015). Jefferson Center for Interprofessional Education (JCIPE) creates TeamSTEPPS® workshops for patient safety

training for students. *Population Health Matters, 28*(3), 3–4.

Gaba, D. M. (2004). The future vision of simulation in health care. *Quality and Safety in Health Care, 13*(Suppl. 1), i2–i10. doi:10.1136/qhc.13.suppl_1.i2

Hayden, J., Smiley, R., Alexander, M., Kardong-Edgren, S., & Jeffries, P. (2014). The NCSBN National Simulation Study: A longitudinal, randomized, controlled study replacing clinical hours with simulation in prelicensure nursing education. *Journal of Nursing Regulation, 5*(2), s4–s41.

Institute for Healthcare Improvement. (2004). 100,000 Lives Campaign. Available at http://www.ihi.org

Institute of Medicine. (2001). *Crossing the quality chasm: A new health system for the 21st century.* Washington, DC: National Academies Press.

Interprofessional Education Collaborative Expert Panel. (2011). *Core competencies for interprofessional collaborative practice: Report of an expert panel.* Washington, DC: Interprofessional Education Collaborative.

Jeffries, P. (2005). A framework for designing, implementing, and evaluating simulations used as teaching strategies in nursing. *Nursing Education Perspectives, 26*(2), 96–103.

Joint Commission. (2008). Sentinel Event Alert: Behaviors that undermine a culture of safety. Retrieved June 7, 2016, from http://www.jointcommission.org/assets/1/18/sea_40.PDF

Jones, K., Skinner, A., High, R., & Reiter-Palmon, R. (2013). A theory-driven, longitudinal evaluation of the impact of team training on safety culture in 24 hospitals. *Quality and Safety in Health Care, 2*(5), 394–404.

King, H. B., Battles, J., Baker, D. P., Alonso, A., Salas, E., Webster, J., et al. (2008). TeamSTEPPS™: Team strategies and tools to enhance performance and patient safety. In K. Henriksen, J. B. Battles, M. A. Keyes, & M. L. Grady (Eds.), *Advances in patient safety: New directions and alternative approaches* (Vol. 3: Performance and Tools, pp. 5–20). Rockville, MD: Agency for Healthcare Research and Quality.

Kirsh, D., & Boysen, P. (2010). Changing the culture in medical education to teach patient safety. *Health Affairs, 29*(9), 1600–1604.

Kohn, L., Corrigan, J., & Donaldson, M. (1999). *To err is human: Building a safer health system. A report of the Committee on Quality of Health Care in America.* Washington, DC: National Academies Press.

Leonard, M., Graham, S., & Bonacum, D. (2004). The human factor: The critical importance of effective teamwork and communication in providing safe care. *Quality and Safety in Health Care, 13*(Suppl. 1), i85–i90.

Meakim, C., Boese, T., Decker, S., Franklin, A. E., Gloe, D., Lioce, L., et al. (2013). Standards of best practice: Simulation standard I: Terminology. *Clinical Simulation in Nursing, 9*(Suppl. 6), s3–s11. doi:10.1016/j.ecns. 2013.04.001

Meyer, G., Denham, C. R., Battles, J. (2010). Safe Practices for Better Healthcare—2010 Update: A Consensus Report. National Quality Forum. Washington, D.C.

National Council of State Boards of Nursing. (2005). *Clinical instruction in prelicensure nursing programs* (Position Paper). Retrieved June 7, 2016, from https://www.ncsbn.org/ Final_Clinical_Instr_Pre_Nsg_programs.pdf

National League for Nursing. (2001). http:// www.nln.org/docs/default-source/ professional-development-programs/ white-paper-symposium-ipe-in-healthcare- simulation-2013-(pdf).pdf?sfvrsn=0

Nickerson, M., Morrison, B., & Pollard, M. (2011). Simulation in nursing staff development: A concept analysis. *Journal for Nurses in Staff Development, 27*(2), 81–89.

O'Daniel, M., & Rosenstein A. H. (2008). Professional communication and team collaboration. *Patient safety and quality: An evidence-based handbook for nurses.* Rockville, MD: Agency for Healthcare Research and Quality. http://www.ncbi.nlm. nih.gov/books/NBK2637p.3

Orasanu, J., & Fischer, U. (2008). Improving healthcare communication: Lessons from the flightdeck. In C. Nemeth (Ed.), *Improving healthcare team communication: Building on lessons from aviation and aerospace* (pp. 23–46). Burlington, VT: Ashgate Publishing.

Rudolph, J. W., Simon, R., Dufresne, R. L., & Raemer, D. B. (2006). There's no such thing as "nonjudgmental" debriefing: A theory and method for debriefing with good judgment. *Simulation in Healthcare: The Journal of the Society for Medical Simulation, 1*(1), 49–55.

Rudolph, J. W., Simon, R., Rivard, P., Dufresne, R. L., & Raemer, D. B. (2007). Debriefing with good judgment: Combining rigorous feedback with genuine inquiry. *Anesthesiology Clinics, 25*(2), 361–376. doi:10.1016/j.anclin

Studdert, D. M., Brennan, T. A., & Thomas, E. J. (2002). What have we learned since the Harvard Medical Practice Study? In M. M. Rosenthal & K. M. Sutcliffe (Eds.), *Medical error: What do we know? What do we do?* (pp. 3–34). San Francisco: Jossey-Bass.

Sutcliffe, K., Lewton, E., & Rosenthal, M. (2004). Communication failures: An insidious contributor to medical mishaps. *Academic Medicine Issue, 79*(2), 186–194.

Ulrich, B., & Kear, T. (2014). Patient safety and patient safety culture: Foundations of excellent health care delivery. *Nephrology Nursing Journal, 41*(5), 447.

Weaver, S., Lubomksi, L., Wilson, R., Pfoh, E., Martinez, K., & Dy, S. (2013). Promoting a culture of safety as a patient safety strategy: A systematic review. *Annals of Internal Medicine, 158*(5), 369–374.

Wilhaus, J., Palaganas, J., Manos, J., Anderson, J., Cooper, A., Jeffries, P., et al. (2012). *Interprofessional education and healthcare simulation symposium.* Retrieved June 7, 2016, from http://www.nln.org/docs/default- source/professional-development-programs/ white-paper-symposium-ipe-in-healthcare- simulation-2013-(pdf).pdf?sfvrsn=0

World Health Organization. (2010). *Framework for action on interprofessional education and collaborative practice.* Geneva, Switzerland: Author. Available at http://apps.who.int/ iris/bitstream/10665/70185/1/WHO_HRH_ HPN_10.3_eng.pdf

10

Interprofessional Education: The International Context

Anne R. Bavier, PhD, RN, FAAN

The purpose of this chapter is to provide a conceptual framework for considering interprofessional education (IPE) within the international context. Throughout this book, the rich, informative discussions of both the why and how of interprofessional practice and education provide the basis for considering IPE within the international arena. In a world where people, disease, and information travel at lightning speeds, nurses must recognize that they live and work within the dynamics of international forces. Never again can any country be the isolationist that George Washington envisioned for a successful society. Today's world is all about international perspectives, and IPE is really no different. In fact, educators do a disservice to students if they do not alert them to international milieu as the broadest dimensions of successfully living within society.

Educators must consider their obligation within the international healthcare arena. Thinking about international perspectives in healthcare, it is clear that multiple agendas and strategies exist, ranging from developing and sharing new knowledge in international clinical investigations, presentations of data and theories, and publications that deliberately strive to bring multiple national perspectives before a broad audience (i.e., *Cancer Nursing: An International Journal for Cancer Care* and multiple publications of Sigma Theta Tau International Inc.). Others look at cultural perspectives that influence individuals who become clients within our U.S. healthcare system and at international differences in healthcare policies.

The ranks of those who conduct science and share findings internationally are limited primarily to those whose investigations advance knowledge about diseases, disorders and conditions experienced across borders. Other international efforts are more concrete—the provision of services to improve the human condition. Perhaps, the incalculable number of service efforts far exceeds the scientific ones. Operation Smile©, the Mercy Ships©, CARE©, and countless mission-oriented expeditions by faith-based communities and the international work of other not-for-profit groups all point to a massive effort of people to serve others. In the United States (and elsewhere), this approach is augmented by numerous colleges and universities "adopting" communities to focus multiple service-oriented projects that may include sanitation, engineering, and land conservation, as well as health education and care provided by students who are engaged in innumerable academic programs. Inevitably, the educators include learners as they embark on service. In addition, in nursing, there are increasing calls for study-abroad experiences, where students perform clinical services and interact directly with other nations' providers and citizens, as evidenced by the National League for Nursing's publication of *Global Service-Learning in Nursing* (McKinnon & Fitzpatrick, 2011), which contains detailed strategies for faculty and administrators to create and sustain such programs. It becomes imperative, therefore, to examine international health professions education within this complex, evolving IPE and service milieu.

OPERATIONAL DEFINITION: INTERNATIONAL PROJECTS

Traditional definitions of the term *international* focus on the joining of ideas, products, or services from more than one nation (Merriam-Webster, 2016). Consider, for example, that daily life is influenced by international businesses, such as McDonald's Corporation or Bayer Corporation. For instance, nursing publications increasingly are managed by international corporations, and many manufacturers who make manikins and other teaching aids are international companies.

In academia, *international* frequently refers to study abroad or sabbatical exchanges of professors with other lands. There are projects that can have many forms in the global context. They can be multisite studies, activities to provide safe water (e.g., digging wells), or training a specific workforce. Among the most compelling in healthcare are projects that prepare local healthcare workers to serve their nations (Murray, 2011) or directly provide services that range from basic immunizations and primary care to those that provide specialty medical care, such as surgical procedures, or investigations to stop ravaging infectious diseases, such as Ebola.

International projects are defined here as a service-oriented activity in a nation different from the one of those who organize the initiative, with the collaboration and concurrence of the receiving or host community. Note that the collaboration and participation of the *host* community is a requisite. International projects can be led by individuals in any nation who conduct an activity in another nation. There is no specification of whether or not it is composed of a single or multiple disciplines. Therefore, a basic tenet is that international projects are not intended to be imposed on a community; rather, they meet a community need, which the project can relieve or adjudicate. This ingredient in international projects underscores the purpose of improving the world as an underlying goal, which many consider social responsibility. This collaboration often is evident in organizational strategies of simultaneously doing numerous international projects in a specific community, or returning to the same community often. Hence, international project participants can be individuals from a variety of professions that may or may not include healthcare.

TENETS OF INTERPROFESSIONAL EDUCATION

In considering international projects and IPE, a quick (not comprehensive) list of the relevant features of IPE is necessary. Traditionally, IPE exists when a team of faculty from multiple disciplines come together to create joint learning experiences for students, usually of their respective disciplines. Previous chapters have noted that when creating IPE learning opportunities, faculty first gain insight and understanding of the various participating disciplines and jointly explore how those disciplinary perspectives unfold in the learning situation contemplated for the IPE experience. Together, the faculty explore in depth the roles and responsibilities that each discipline could and should contribute. The faculty team becomes a role model that allows the situation to determine which discipline provides the leadership. There are no predetermined hierarchical arrangements. Students are invited to the learning experiences and learn together using a variety of pedagogical approaches, such as simulation, debriefing, or unfolding case studies. The expected outcome is that learners gain knowledge about their roles, responsibilities of other disciplines, and experience faculty interactions that demonstrate respect and understanding of other disciplines. Kendall et al. (2008) stress the importance of IPE if practice is to develop true and effective teamwork. They further emphasize that academic institutions can support reflective practice and research into IPE and its outcomes to strengthen the strategies.

As described previously, pedagogical differences, scheduling logistics, resource allocation, and philosophical differences related to hierarchical relationships and authority (Kendall, et al., 2008; De Los Santos, McFarlin, & Martin, 2014) have already been established as barriers to IPE. Personal bias of faculty members toward other professions can be a barrier as well. Unwillingness to embrace the new ways of teaching and learning may further complicate the experiences (Kendall et al., 2008).

The focus of IPE is the learner; patient foci are facilitators of the learning outcomes, not the method's primary purpose. In this regard, IPE resembles discipline-specific education. Clearly, patients and communities benefit from the presence and interventions of the learners and their faculty. This is particularly true in traditional health professions education clinical practice experiences, where faculty members would not provide care or even be present, except for their teaching obligations. This is a highly relevant point for this discussion, because international projects should be built around a service-learning orientation.

SERVICE-LEARNING: AN IMPORTANT EDUCATIONAL STRATEGY

Major efforts on defining and describing service-learning occurred in the 1990s, with continuing refinement over time. Bringle and Hatcher (1996) defined *service-learning* as "a credit-bearing educational experience in which students participate in an organized service activity that meets identified community needs....This experience adds depth to the learning that is associated with stated course goals. To them, the process also results in 'an enhanced sense of civic responsibility'" (p. 222). They note that this is not necessarily skill-based learning, such as in a practica or internship. Rather, they emphasize the importance of a credit-based learning experience for students, because service-learning is another educational strategy to achieve course objectives. Others add that the experience strengthens the host communities where the activities occur and that it is the partnerships between the educational institution and the communities that make the system work. It is a mutually beneficial or reciprocal relationship between the academic institution and community (Seifer, 1998; Bailey, Carpenter, & Harrington, 2002). Students apply classroom knowledge in real-world situations, thus experiencing the role of contributing citizens (Seifer, 1998). Students need to know what is to be accomplished (the service) and what is to be learned (the course credit linkage). But service-learning is different from volunteerism. In efforts to give services to underserved populations both within the United States and in international projects, volunteerism is a situation where the patient comes first, not the learner (Wilson, Merry, & Franz, 2012). Service-learning values both the gains of students and the patients *equally.* International experiences often are arranged for learners as a part of a voluntary group's service. Faith-based organizations and service-oriented groups are typical sponsoring organizations. Faculty who embrace such work often volunteer their time and invite students to accompany the group. The purpose of the volunteer work is service, not necessarily the students' learning. The focus often is entirely on meeting the needs of the partner community, such as providing health screening or educational services. Students are present to provide part of the service, and any learning is a secondary outcome. These volunteer service experiences may not be service-learning, because they lack the reflection and academic development inherent in service-learning. As discussed previously, volunteer groups often have many types of health professionals, theologians, and laypeople but may not actually be an interprofessional team. For example, a surgical team may work in the customary fashion of specified roles and hierarchy that would be found in any U.S. institution, whereas engineers work on sanitation issues in their customary manner. Thus, parallel activities may be the best approach to accomplish the service goals.

Previously, Honnett and Poulsen (1989) articulated principles of good practice when combining service and learning (later called *service-learning*). Among these principles are that the activities and actions are being done for the common good with clear service and learning goals. The principles include that community partners' defined needs match the scope of service activities proposed and that those partnerships are sustained over time (not merely a one-time interaction). The host community must define its needs (not the service providers), which can change over time. Critical reflection by learners is a central tenet of the principles. This means that the learners will experience consequences of their actions; they are not observers (Honnett & Poulsen, 1989). Here the community is specifically the one receiving the benefits of the service in the service-learning model. Further, community can be defined by the group itself or geographically. Both perspectives are relevant to international work. The community must work closely with the education group and have joint responsibilities and accountability. It is a joint effort, or partnership (Seifer, 1998). In defining community, for example, the partnership could be established with a specific village or town in another nation. At other times, prevailing needs may surpass the town or village and the community becomes a population, such as those needing vaccines or surgeries to repair head and neck malformations in children. The partnerships then form around a network of host entities. Regardless, leaders of those communities are vital to successful service-learning relationships. It is therefore imperative that nursing students engaged in these types of international interprofessional service-learning relationships understand that the team leader is often the host (community) leader.

The pedagogy of service-learning involves the role of faculty as a facilitator of learning, is different from the traditional role of controller of knowledge. A key construct of service-learning is that of reflection by learners. As in IPE, faculty guide reflection through multiple techniques, such as diaries and discussion groups, and they link the course knowledge, skills, and concepts to the experience of the learner. Moral and social issues and the individual's roles and responsibilities also typically arise in the reflection exercises. Numerous benefits of the service-learning strategy are described in the literature. Service-learning is viewed as a way in which academic institutions fulfill their responsibilities to society, beyond the preparation of "learned individuals." Faculty and students are both seen as beneficiaries of the processes, as they gain knowledge of a community, its needs, cultural perspectives, and the context of others' existence. Students' reflections show development in areas of understanding of civic responsibility to engage in service (Stallwood & Groh, 2011).

The nature of the partnership makes the community members teachers as well. It is the interaction between the community members and learners that provides the fodder for gaining insights into the culture and its habits (Bavier, 2012). Trust between and among the receiving community leaders and the service team is a must. Ventres and Wilson (2015) refer to this as the bidirectional scope of international projects. As Marcus, Taylor, Hormann, Walker, and Carroll (2011) modified service-learning as community-based participatory research, they remarked that trust is imperative for the service and learning outcomes. They further note that frequent meetings between the academic team and community stakeholders build the relationship and focus on the needs of the community. Therefore, service-learning often advances the academic institutions' commitment to preparation of individuals to work within culturally diverse settings and to advance learners' understanding and competency in managing populations and peoples from communities where poverty and ethnic diversity are dominant. Siantz (2008) notes that in organizations seeking to improve cultural competence, risk taking often is necessary, taking faculty out of their comfort zones. Mason and Anderson (2007) state that the building of capacity for international learning experiences requires mutual trust, which encompasses tolerating ambiguity that may be taking risks about the unknowns. Service-learning as an action-oriented approach coupled with reflection and multiple faculty techniques designed to advance students' insight are seen as major advantages of developing cultural competency. These insights are even more powerful when they are magnified through the lens of other members of the service-learning team. For the nursing student, gaining this perspective can have a profound effect on his or her praxis.

INTERNATIONAL SERVICE-LEARNING

Due largely to the challenges of orchestrating education in another country, American health professions education endeavors often adopt the service-learning approach. International practical experiences are sought for numerous reasons, most notably the importance of preparing graduates to live and function in multicultural environments and to increase awareness of other health systems and perspectives in care organization and delivery.

McKinnon and Fealy (2011) address the appropriateness of a service-learning model for international education. They delineate core principles of international service-learning as compassion, curiosity, courage, collaboration, creativity, capacity building, and competence. *Compassion* refers to both faculty passion to prepare the next generation of nurses with a global perspective and service orientation, and students developing recognition of social responsibility. *Curiosity* is described as the energy to learn about other cultures and issues in global health, and stems from faculty curiosity in those areas. *Courage* to embark on an unfamiliar journey is requisite among planners, faculty, and learners. Because service-learning is a partnership with communities and academia, *collaboration* means that there is no hierarchical relationship; norms for the partnership are established by the group itself. These partnerships are sustained over time. *Creativity* is innovation and reflects the uncharted territory of the partnerships that requires new solutions. Service-learning, particularly in the global context, is not intended to cultivate a dependent relationship of either partner. Rather, the service-learning is to *build capacity* that builds *competence* in all.

Kollar and Ailinger (2002) report an international cultural immersion experience with undergraduate and graduate nursing students in Nicaragua. Based at a university that had been placing students in a 2-week experience for several years, the authors contacted 12 alumni and asked them about the long-term impact of their experience. These alumni reported a positive influence on how they see clients and interact with those from other cultures. Awareness of the Hispanic culture and a more realistic approach to planning and evaluation were noted as well. Personal growth influenced career changes, such as working in a public health clinic and the Peace Corps and respect for what clinicians in Nicaragua achieve with comparatively few resources. Kollar and Ailinger (2002) concluded that the experience left a mark in the minds and hearts of participants that was indelible.

Bentley and Ellison (2007) remarked that international service-learning offers a unique opportunity because students work in another culture, requiring their adaptation. They developed a credit-bearing course for senior nursing students in their last semester, with significant pretrip planning with the local partner organization. Their experience focused on women's health in an Ecuadorian village that was professionally staffed by the community partner. The partner's knowledge of the local community's needs and strategies made the planning and execution effective, although they note that both planning and execution phases were time intensive. Through survey instruments and students' written narratives, they report that students gained cultural competency. The experience was with a small number of students who only spent a week in Ecuador, but it demonstrates the key element of cooperation (McKinnon & Fealy, 2011).

Kiely (2004) noted that many report findings of positive outcomes immediately after an international service-learning experience. He conducted a longitudinal case study of 22 students who had a similar international service-learning experience with an emphasis on social justice. He used a framework that seeks to learn about the students' transformational learning, in contrast to instrumental learning, which uses the individual's current frame of reference and adds knowledge. Perspective transformational learning changes the frame of reference—the underlying assumptions through which the world is viewed. Such learning changes the perspectives to ones that are more relevant to the experience. The findings of intensive interviews of these program alumni from a service-learning trip to Nicaragua revealed that all had experienced perspective transformation as emerging global consciousness. The ongoing challenge for returnees is to find ways to act on those changes—what Kiely (2004) terms the *chameleon complex.* Kiely concluded that there is a need to find ways that returnees can engage in relevant social action, and he raises the issue of the ethical challenge to faculty who promote perspective transformations without providing the structural guidance for learners to meaningfully engage their new insights.

Ventres and Wilson (2015) are both physicians and anthropologists whose international service-learning trips provided insight into attitudes that can be nurtured in such experiences, as well as problematic attitudes that can develop. The focus is individuals traveling from highly developed nations to developing ones. They describe *open-mindedness* as an attitude that allows individual participants to note how others interact and how various skill mixes of professionals contribute to the services provided. *Humility,* another attitude, recognizes that the human condition and its challenges are shared by all, not merely those who experience the suffering. The authors differentiate *generosity* as an attitude, which allows people as individuals and as professionals to experience the "give and take" of situations. In other words, it is a reciprocal relationship, whereas altruism is giving, not receiving, in the relationships. *Patience* is the fourth attitude described, and it is the recognition that the fast pace often present in highly developed nations typically does not exist in developing ones. In contrast to professional work in highly developed nations with boundless resources, *excellence* is an attitude acknowledging that quality must be considered in terms of resources available and cultural dynamics.

The potential "attitudinal traps" described by Ventres and Wilson (2015) add a rich perspective for consideration in international service-learning. *Arrogance* is the antithesis of humility and relates to feeling superior, or better, than others. Interestingly, the authors note that the extensive, effusive thanks offered by hosts can inadvertently foster arrogance. *Hegemony* is domination. In the international service-learning experience, it is an attitude of visitors from highly developed nations dominating the situation, without the sensitivity to culture and other factors. Another attitude that hinders full success of international service-learning is that of *indebtedness,* which is closely related to domination in that those from high-resource nations believe that others should be especially grateful for things given to them, such as surgical dressings or medications. When visitors from a highly developed nation see a segment of need and provide services without consideration for sustaining the program or future needs for cooperation, the authors designate this as *balkanization.* Finally, the authors caution against using a friendship network to take services to developing nations without building the cooperation and partnerships with the actual host. This power by proxy or "buddy" approach underscores the need for a basic tenet of service-learning—the significant collaboration and partnership between groups. Wilson, Merry, and Franz (2012) note that there is also a danger of promoting dependency on the international project team rather than fostering sustainable communities.

International education programs may use a service-learning approach with generally seen positive short-term (end of experience) and long-term changes in perspectives, although few studies are identified by this author to document these outcomes. Data are primarily qualitative analyses of narratives or interviews with program alumni. Repeated rigorous mixed method research on outcomes needs to be undertaken. However, institutional pressures to conduct study-abroad learning courses and a calling to meet academia's service mission provide confidence that international experiences for undergraduate and graduate students will continue. That said, there is a place for consideration of international, interprofessional service-learning.

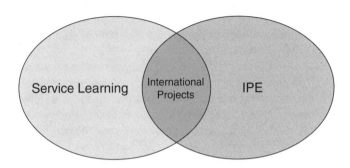

FIGURE 10.1 In the international arena, there is a clear overlap between service-learning and IPE (Bavier, 2012).

THE MODEL: INTERPROFESSIONAL EDUCATION IN THE INTERNATIONAL ARENA

Conceptually, service-learning and IPE can be viewed as distinct conceptual and operational paradigms. However, in the international arena, there is a clear overlap because of the necessity to employ the strategies of service-learning (particularly that of collaboration) to achieve a viable, meaningful learning experience (Figure 10.1). Successful international projects can employ and develop characteristics of service-learning to enhance their effectiveness.

In particular, the international projects should use many techniques and guiding principles from both the IPE and service-learning domains. The host community is viewed as a partner and collaborator in determining priority needs and services to be provided. The leaders of the host community can represent many health disciplines but do not need to exactly replicate those doing the service-learning. Part of the education experience is to understand how various cultural groups organize their professional and lay resources to achieve goals. The long-term relationships are built with the host community and typically involve repeated international experiences for the IPE team members. Although the host community participants and IPE team members change over time, most can expect some constant participants to build on previous interactions and projects to produce relevant new collaborations. Awarding academic credits ties the service experience to a knowledge component and allows for meaningful use of reflection and other techniques that are intended to enhance the personal and professional growth of the learner. The organizing faculty is an interprofessional team that uses situational leadership to determine its priorities and actions. As the community partnership evolves and service projects change, different disciplines may become leaders of the faculty team. This distribution of responsibilities over time benefits the other faculty members and learners as people immerse themselves in different approaches and strategies. All faculty members and the community partners are teachers of all learners. Discipline-specific interactions are only to enhance the understanding of the interprofessional team. The emphasis on learning is equal to service in all elements of the international project, supporting and underscoring the feasibility of deliberately merging the two approaches.

De Los Santos et al. (2014) discussed an IPE sequence required in nursing, medicine, social work, and public health curricula. Students work on an interprofessional

---

BOX 10.1

International Interprofessional Exemplar

Universitas 21 (U21) (www.U21health.org) used a summer experiences model constructed around a topic important in the international health arena, and the U21 experiences were highly relevant in a global context. The academic institution provided the faculty team, and faculty from various health disciplines could accompany their students and participate. The first program was offered by the University of Auckland in summer 2014, entitled "Substance Misuse Studies: A Harm Reduction Approach." Twenty-six students from nine disciplines and 12 countries participated in the 2-week course. Course experiences included visiting clinical facilities and working in interprofessional teams of students and faculty to devise interventions for the subject population. Overall, students rated the program as very successful and valuable. Scholarships reduced the costs, which students appreciated.

In summer 2015, Tecnologico de Monterrey hosted a program on the topics of vulnerability and low-budget healthcare. Fifteen students representing nine countries and nine disciplines attended the 2-week program. Experiences included working with the elderly, interprofessional teams of students, and faculty members and development of interventions. Participation and projects were graded and credit awarded by the host university.

The 2016 program will be offered at Pontificia Universidad Catolica de Chile and will focus on early critical windows of prevention intervention. Clinical observations in an antepartum center are designed to teach learners to identify those early developmental windows of possible intervention.

---

team visiting families in a designated geographical area. The needs of the families determine the purposes and interventions for each home visit (which occur at least quarterly). Preparation for home visits was coordinated through attendance at an interprofessional workshop, and faculty served as members of the disciplines participating and supervised the students. The project employed key principles of service-learning (e.g., definition of issues based on families' needs), collaboration of community agencies in identifying potential families, and the continuity of the teams in the community over time. Box 10.1 provides an international interprofessional exemplar.

CONCLUSION

In this chapter, the unique domain of health education in the international arena was explored as an integration of the characteristics of IPE and service-learning. Through such combination, nursing and all health disciplines can move from their discipline-specific foci to a broader perspective in preparing future health providers. The goal to advance the human condition worldwide taps the social responsibilities of individuals and institutions. As advances in technology, people's mobility, and expediential growth of knowledge occur, information exchange mandates that we foster learners' awareness and participation in global health issues. As educators, we can prepare students for the interprofessional practices that employ the best services to gain the desired outcomes. IPE can be coupled with service-learning to provide robust, meaningful experiences for host communities, faculties, and students in the international program setting.

References

Bailey, P. A., Carpenter, D. R., & Harrington, P. (2002). Theoretical foundations of service-learning in nursing education. *Journal of Nursing Education, 41*(10), 433–436.

Bavier, A. R. (2012). International-interprofessional health sciences education: A U21 model for consideration. *Universitas 21 Health Sciences.* Retrieved June 8, 2016, from http://U21health.org/summer-school

Bentley, R., & Ellison, K. J. (2007). Increasing cultural competence in nursing through international service-learning experiences. *Nurse Educator, 32*(5), 207–211.

Bringle, R. G., & Hatcher, J. A. (1996). Implementing service learning in higher education. *Journal of Higher Education, 67*(2), 221–239.

De Los Santos, S., McFarlin, C. D., & Martin, L. (2014). Interprofessional education and service learning: A model for the future of health professions education. *Journal of Interprofessional Care, 28*(4), 374–375.

Honnett, E. P., & Poulsen, S. J. (1989). *Principles of good practice for combining service and learning.* Racine, WA: Johnson Foundation. Available at http://digitalcommons. unomaha.edu/slceguides/27

Kendall, H., Jarvis-Selinger, S., Borduas, F., Frank, B., Hall, P., Handfield-Jones, R., et al. (2008). Making interprofessional education work: The strategic roles of the academy. *Academic Medicine, 83*(10), 934–940.

Kiely, R. (2004). A chameleon with a complex: Searching for transformation in international service-learning. *Michigan Journal of Community Service Learning, 10*(2), 5–20.

Kollar, S. J., & Ailinger, R. L. (2002). International clinical experiences: Long-term impact on students. *Nurse Educator, 27*(1), 28–31.

Marcus, M. T., Taylor, W. C., Hormann, M. D., Walker, T., & Carroll, D. (2011). Linking service-learning with community-based participatory research: An interprofessional course for health professional students. *Nursing Outlook, 59*(1), 47–54.

Mason, C. H., & Anderson, M. C. (2007). Developing an international learning experience in the Gambia, West Africa: The rewards and challenges of a complex partnership. *Journal of Cultural Diversity, 14*(1), 35–42.

McKinnon, T. H., & Fealy, G. (2011). Core principles for developing global service-learning programs in nursing. *Nursing Education Perspectives, 32*(2), 95–101.

McKinnon, T. H., & Fitzpatrick, J. (Eds.). 2011. *Global service-learning in nursing.* New York: National League for Nursing.

Merriam-Webster. (2016). Merriam-Webster dictionary. Available at: www.merriam-webster.com/dictionary/international

Murray, J. P. (2011). *Educating health professionals in low-resource countries: A global approach.* New York: Springer.

Seifer, S. D. (1998). Service-learning: community-campus partnerships for health professions education. *Academic Medicine, 73*(3), 273–277.

Siantz, M. (2008). Leading change in diversity and cultural competence. *Journal of Professional Nursing, 24*(3), 167–171.

Stallwood, L. G., & Groh, C. J. (2011). Service-learning in the nursing curriculum: Are we at the level of evidence-based practice? *Nursing Education Perspectives, 32*(5), 297–301.

Ventres, W. B., & Wilson, C. L. (2015). Beyond ethical and curricular guidelines in global health: Attitudinal development on international service-learning trips. *BMC Medical Education, 15*(68), 1–5.

Wilson, J. W., Merry, S. P., & Franz, W. B. (2012). Rules of engagement: The principles of underserved global health volunteerism. *American Journal of Medicine, 125*(6), 612–617.

Evaluating and Disseminating Interprofessional Education

Kevin J. Lyons, PhD, FASAHP

Carolyn Giordano, PhD

As discussed throughout this book, interprofessional education (IPE) and collaborative practice (CP) is a model that is fast becoming the norm in healthcare due to the rise in the complexity and integrated nature of healthcare. It has become accepted that the needs of patients are often greater than one single health profession can address and requires collaboration on the part of healthcare providers (Freeth, 2001). This growing need for more collaboration has resulted in more attention on the interprofessional practice and education of healthcare professionals (Schofield & Amodeo, 1999). Over the past few years, there has been a cultural shift in training to prepare health professionals. These training programs are now an integral part of the curriculum in many nursing, medical, and health education programs, and they are slowly being integrated into clinical sites. Data suggests that interprofessional care by well-functioning teams results in improved patient outcomes and can be cost effective (Interprofessional Education Collaborative [IPEC] Expert Panel, 2011). As mentioned in Chapter 5, the World Health Organization has recognized this on an international level, asserting that "[a]fter almost 50 years of inquiry, there is now sufficient evidence to indicate that IPE enables effective CP, which in turn optimizes health services, strengthens health systems and improves health outcomes" (World Health Organization, 2010, p. 18). It is important that research in this area continues. Interprofessional models of education and care require that the programs be theoretically based and educationally sound. Conducting rigorous evaluation of these programs will add to the growing body of research, which facilitates the understanding of the most effective ways to prepare students and clinicians to function as members of interprofessional teams. Like any other evaluation process, the goal of measuring the impact of IPE and/or CP programs should be to drive both short- and long-term decision making.

Although evaluation of any project should be an integral part of the planning phase, just determining the results of a program is not enough. Naturally, it is valuable to know how successful a program is, but it is also important to disseminate program evaluation results to build a body of knowledge to support interprofessional care and education. In the literature, some authors make the distinction between *program assessment* and *program evaluation* (Barnstable, 2003, p. 494–495), whereas others use the terms interchangeably.

Both of these rely on the gathering, summarizing, and interpreting of data. Assessment uses these processes to guide future action, whereas evaluation uses them to determine if the action was successful. The steps in the process are the same; it is the purpose that is different. It is important to note that although creating an evaluation plan at the time of program development is important, the ability and willingness to disseminate findings through presentations and publications is equally important.

DEVELOPING AN INTERPROFESSIONAL PROGRAM EVALUATION PLAN

Program evaluation is a systematic process and should be a fundamental part of any project from the beginning. As noted, deciding on how to assess the results of a project should not begin when the program or project has already started. Rather, developing an evaluation plan needs to be an integral part of the total program planning process. Figure 11.1 is an exemplar of an IPE and/or CP program evaluation plan.

Identifying the goals of the project is the first step in its development. Evaluation should be decided at the onset of the project development, and identifying the methods that will be used to evaluate them should be done before the project commences. In deciding an evaluation methodology, it is important to determine what methods, tools, and evaluation processes have been done previously on similar topics. A wide search of the literature that includes nursing and other disciplines should be done, as the amount of research into these areas has expanded exponentially in recent years. Questions that frame an IPE literature search include the following: Have similar projects been done? What were the stated goals of these projects, and how have they been evaluated? What theoretical models have been used, and could these models be used as a guide? Was a

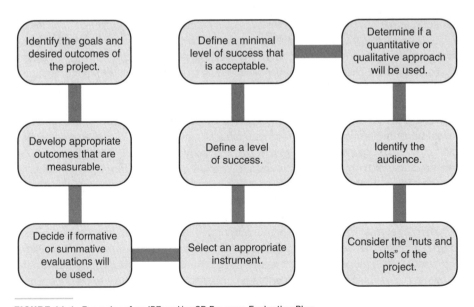

FIGURE 11.1 Exemplar of an IPE and/or CP Program Evaluation Plan.

conceptual model used to frame the project? If so, could that framework be generalizable across multiple situations?

Once the goals of the project have been identified, ensure that they are clear, well defined, and measurable. Identifying how the goals will be measured in the beginning will not only serve as a test of their suitability but also ensure that it will be possible to determine success or failure of the project. If the project goals are too obscure or unclear, it may be impossible to measure them in any meaningful way. For example, "The goal of this project is to teach students about teamwork" is too vague. What about teamwork will be taught? A better goal might be "The goal of this project is to have students understand the 14 characteristics of effective teams." This goal is both clear enough and measureable.

The goals of a project should clearly identify appropriate outcomes. What are the outcomes determining that each particular goal was achieved? Is the program seeking to determine if there is participant satisfaction, knowledge, behavior, achievement, attitudes, or understanding? One popular conceptual model is Kirkpatrick's model. This model lays out a hierarchy of outcomes to help guide the formulation of program evaluation strategies and is discussed in detail in Chapter 2.

Once the goals and outcomes are determined, the next step is to decide if both formative and/or summative evaluations will be needed. Formative evaluations are conducted periodically during a project and provide an indication as to whether the project is "on track" and progressing the way it was intended. These can be valuable in projects that are long term, as they will reveal that something is not proceeding appropriately, which allows for any necessary changes along the way. Formative evaluations can also help test the evaluation strategy to ensure that it is providing the intended information. Summative evaluations are conducted at the end of the project and are the ones that indicate whether or not the program has succeeded in accomplishing its goals. Often, for projects of a relatively brief duration, summative evaluations are all that will be needed. In some long-term educational projects where there are clear segments, the summative evaluation of one segment can act as a formative evaluation for the next segment.

The next step is to identify and select an appropriate measuring instrument. Selecting an appropriate instrument can only be accomplished through a thorough literature review. The literature contains a large number of instruments measuring almost every aspect of interprofessional care and education. Although it is possible to develop an instrument and design it for the specifics of the program being created, it is not recommended because developing a valid and reliable instrument is a time-consuming project all to itself. However, if none of the myriad published instruments fits the programs' goals, developing an instrument might be necessary. Some resources for identifying IPE instruments are outlined in a report by the Canadian Interprofessional Health Collaborative (2012), entitled *An Inventory of Quantitative Tools to Measure Interprofessional Education and Collaborative Practice.* Additional evaluation resources can be found on the National Center for Interprofessional Practice and Education (2015) website (www.nexusipe.org) or in most libraries using the Health and Psychosocial Instruments citation resource. Most instruments are copyrighted and permission is usually required, but authors are generally pleased to grant permission to keep track of how many times the instrument is being utilized.

Once an appropriate instrument has been identified, defining success is the next step. For example, if a quantitative approach is being used, consider what is the minimal level of difference in the outcome measure that is acceptable for the project to be considered a success. If change over time is being measured, then what is the minimal amount of change that will be accepted? If groups are being compared, what will be the accepted statistically significant differences in the measure, or will a certain level of difference be acceptable even though it is not significant? Sometimes the significance level is determined by the sample size. Smaller samples require larger differences to be statistically significant. Most clinical or educational programs have relatively small samples, especially those projects or programs that are just beginning. Most journals look for a statistical significance level at .05 or .01. However, setting a level is a relatively arbitrary decision, and it just means that being wrong 5 percent or 1 percent of the time is acceptable. Therefore, would a significance level at the .10 level be acceptable? Setting this level should be made pragmatically, given the nature of the particular situation or program.

If a qualitative approach is being used, a definition of success might be slightly different. For example, if students are asked to write reflection papers on an interprofessional experience that they have gone through and the plan is to do a content analysis of these papers, a measure of success might be that students identify common points that they all took away from the experience.

Not often considered, but an important issue in planning an evaluation, is knowing the audience. Will the audience be policymakers at your institution, or will it be those who are running the program or students and/or clinicians? Knowing the audience has implications for the questions that are asked and the way the results are presented. Policymakers will want to see overall effectiveness. Was the project a success? Additionally, they may not be concerned with the details of each part of the project. Those running the project will be interested in overall success as well, but they will also be concerned with the success of each component of the project. The student and/or clinician will be interested in how the program was presented and whether the program helped them understand interprofessional practice and education. In addition, the nature of the audience has implications for the level or outcome measurement plan. For example, if the dean or president is putting resources into the program, he or she will want to know how successful the project is in terms of how well it is meeting the institution's IPE goals. The program developers will be concerned about overall goals but will also be interested in the outcomes of each of the projects that were implemented.

The final step in the creation of IPE programs and initiatives is the cost of administration and the amount of analysis that will be needed. Consider if the evaluation can be done by the program developers or if an outside evaluator will need to be hired and what resources and time are available. These are all critical elements of a successful evaluation plan and will determine the feasibility of conducting an accurate and unbiased evaluation.

COMPONENTS OF AN EVALUATION PLAN

In addition to the steps described earlier, there are several other components of an effective evaluation plan. The plan should have a systematic framework. Four sections typically included in the systematic plan of evaluation include purpose, methods, instruments, and evaluation strategy.

The *purpose* section should identify the reason for conducting the evaluation and describe the overall structure of the plan. This would include the goals of the project; the questions that need to be answered; and possibly the theoretical or conceptual model, such as the Kirkpatrick model, that can be used.

In the *methods* section, the "what," "who," "when," and "how" questions should be identified. In other words, what will be measured? Who is the target audience? When will the data be collected, and how will this be accomplished?

The *instruments* section should provide a description of the data collection instruments and reasons for selecting the specific instrument, including why it is the best instrument to use and the reliability and validity measurements.

Finally, the *evaluation strategy* section should contain a description of how the data will be evaluated. If a quantitative assessment is being conducted, what statistical methods will be used? If a qualitative assessment, how will that data be assessed? If a mixed method approach, then the strategies listed earlier would be combined and the order in which they will be carried out should be stated.

IMPORTANT MEASUREMENTS

There are four characteristics that can be used to determine the success of a project: attitudes, knowledge or skills, behaviors, and effectiveness. See Figure 11.2.

The most basic level of measuring a program is to study changes in *attitudes*. Attitudes are the basis of behavior, and knowing attitudes can be valuable in formative assessment. If someone has a poor attitude about a program, he or she will tend to behave in a negative manner, and if someone has a good attitude, he or she may behave

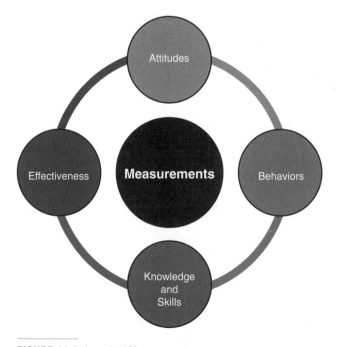

FIGURE 11.2 Important Measurements.

in a more positive manner. In the IPE literature, most of the research and assessment instruments are geared toward attitudinal measurement.

Knowledge or skills would be the next level of complexity. An example of how knowledge or skills is important in IPE would be to examine whether, as a result of the project, participants learned new skills that they could apply to their practice. Are they more knowledgeable about the components of teamwork? Although the evaluation of knowledge gained through an interprofessional experience can usually be assessed accurately through knowledge questions on a posttest, many studies of knowledge and skills learned rely on self-report measures. This can be cause for some concern. The results of self-report measures should be viewed with caution. Individuals can claim that they have increased their skill levels in certain areas or that they are more knowledgeable about a topic, but this might not be the case. It is best to try to obtain more objective measures if possible, such as a return demonstration. Nevertheless, knowledge and skills are important variables to assess, because without them changes in behaviors would not be possible.

It means little if someone has become more knowledgeable, or that he or she has increased skill in an area, but does not use the knowledge and skill in practice. Therefore, *behaviors* are at the next level of complexity. Although there is less current research on this element, many evaluators are now looking at the area more closely. The most effective ways to assess behaviors are through observing teams in action. Those knowledgeable about IPE, possibly using observation instruments, can identify the extent to which members of a team are behaving. A second possible way to assess team behaviors is to interview patients with whom the team has interacted.

Finally, there are measures of *effectiveness*. Is there a relationship between effective team behavior and outcomes? This is the most important level of evaluation. Outcomes are specific measurable things, such as cost, patient safety, patient satisfaction, readmission rates, or length of stay. In the Institute of Medicine (2013) report *Measuring the Impact of Interprofessional Education on Collaborative Practice and Patient Outcomes,* the question has been raised as to whether or not IPE affects patient, population, and health system outcomes. Clearly, this is the area in which there is the greatest need for research and evaluation. Data on the correlation between IPE and patient outcomes is probably the most difficult to collect but arguably is the most valuable. Examining this relationship would require a well-designed, complex study in conjunction with a close working relationship among educators, those in the healthcare delivery system, and often with representatives from a broad array of disciplines, such as economics and health services research. These studies are usually not appropriate for the evaluation of a single interprofessional curriculum, as education is only one piece of this complex puzzle. In addition, these studies are expensive and time consuming and require a team of experts in research.

EVALUATION DESIGNS

Research can be categorized as quantitative, qualitative, or a mix of both approaches. Mixed methods research is common and generally refers to research that employs "both qualitative and quantitative approaches or methods in a single study or program of inquiry" (Tashakkori & Creswell, 2007, p. 4). Both quantitative and qualitative approaches

---

BOX 11.1

Example Research Designs for Evaluation of Interprofessional Education and/or Collaborative Practice Projects

Quantitative
- Surveys
- Structured interviews
- Structured observations
- Randomized clinical trials

Qualitative
- Case studies
- Semistructured interviews
- Unstructured interviews
- Focus groups
- Participant observation

Mixed Method Approaches
- Combination of surveys and focus groups
- Surveys with written response

---

can provide valuable data to assess a program. Quantitative research seeks to produce measurable numerical data to support a hypothesis, and approaches consist of such things as surveys, structured observations, and randomized clinical trials. Qualitative data uncovers opinions and helps us understand the causes of a phenomenon. Approaches could be interviews, focus groups, or unstructured observations. Often, the most powerful approach is when these methods are mixed together, conducting a survey first and examining the outcomes in a deeper fashion through focus groups, interviews, or observations. Scholars have discussed that research on IPE needs to include more longitudinal mixed method studies (Freeth, Hammick, Koppel, Reeves, & Barr, 2002; Humphris & Hean, 2004; Pollard & Miers, 2008). Stone (2006) argues that "traditional, control group experimental designs may not be adequate, appropriate or reasonable as a sole means of evaluating interprofessional education" (p. 260). As with any research, the choice of method depends on the question being asked. Box 11.1 presents the three general categories of design, with examples of each.

RESEARCH DESIGNS AND EVALUATING INTERPROFESSIONAL EDUCATION

Types of Quantitative Evaluation Strategies

Surveys are probably the most often used of the quantitative assessment strategies. They are relatively easy to use and generally less expensive than other methods. A good source to learn about survey design is the Wiley *Handbook of Health Survey Methods* (Johnson, 2014).

As described previously, there are myriad survey instruments cited in the literature that are designed to measure important aspects of interprofessional teamwork. Many of these have high reported levels of reliability and validity. Two scales that fit easily into most IPE initiatives are the Interdisciplinary Education Perception Scale (IEPS) (Luecht, Madsen, Taugher, & Petterson, 1990), an 18-item survey with four subscales that measures attitudes toward IPE, and the Attitudes Toward Health Care Teams Scale (Heinemann, Schmitt, Farrell, & Brallier, 1999), a 20-item survey that assesses an individual's attitude toward teamwork that can be used in evaluating team training programs. In addition, electronic surveys instruments such as Survey Monkey™ are a great evaluation option when only a few questions about the experience are being solicited. These instruments are easy to use and save considerable time and effort by organizing the participant's responses.

Structured interviews are similar to surveys in that they rely on an evaluator asking participants in a project a list of questions related to the outcome of interest, with only predetermined responses possible, such as "rarely," "sometimes," and "often." Although this limits the responses that participants can give, it forces individuals to focus on the specific outcomes that are of interest to the evaluator. An advantage of using structured interviews is that they can be done in person, on the phone, or in a chat room setting. Similarly, a structured observation can be used as another quantitative approach to evaluating IPE programs. A structured observation instrument lays out certain characteristics that should be readily discernible when observing an interprofessional team in action. For example, the *Jefferson Teamwork Observation Guide* (JTOG) (Jefferson Center for Professional Education, 2016) is one easy-to-use instrument that directs individuals to look for certain behaviors from members of a team. This short guide contains examples of five critical components of effective teamwork. These components were derived from the literature on teamwork and are matched to the Interprofessional Education Collaborative (IPEC) Core Competencies. The IPEC Core Competencies have been discussed in detail in many of the previous chapters. The components are roles and responsibilities, communication, values and ethics, and teamwork. Currently, the JTOG has been modified to include the patient and the patient's caregiver (family member and/or loved one), a version that surveys the "real-time" patient experience with the healthcare provider team.

Randomized clinical trials are the most sophisticated of the quantitative approaches. These are clinical studies where volunteer participants with comparable characteristics are randomly assigned to different test groups to compare the efficacy of a particular approach. They are considered the gold standard of scientific research but are expensive and difficult to carry out. Although there have been a few randomized controlled trials addressing the effectiveness of IPE programs, research on the effectiveness of interprofessional interventions is often criticized because of the relative lack of this approach (Reeves, Perrier, Goldman, Freeth, & Zwarenstein, 2013).

Types of Qualitative Evaluation Strategies

Qualitative assessment strategies are becoming more and more accepted in the research community. They run from very simple observation strategies to those requiring major investments in time and money. However, in terms of project evaluation of interprofessional projects, some of the relatively simple ones are probably the most appropriate. Case studies are usually in-depth investigations of a single individual. In rare instances, they can be used to describe the workings of a group. They are often more valuable to use in a team training exercise. For example, a case study of a particular patient can be used to show how the knowledge of members of different disciplines can be used to develop a plan of care. Likewise, semistructured and unstructured interviews are similar to structured interviews, with the exception that more latitude is given to the participants. The questions may be similar, but the participants are asked to explain the answer to the question rather than forced to give predetermined responses. Their answer often results in the interviewer asking more probing questions that are suggested by the initial answers, thereby allowing for a more detailed description than possible with a structured interview. These probing questions often have the added value of unearthing new ideas not intended by the initial set of questions. Focus groups are being used more often in learning about the experience of participants in programs of an interprofessional nature. This approach was initially developed for use in marketing research but is now used as a research tool in many other areas, such as education and healthcare. It is a meeting of a group of 7 to 12 individuals knowledgeable about a situation led by an interviewer skilled in conducting a group process. It is similar to conducting a semistructured interview with a group of people, whereby the interviewer uses a list of questions related to the topic area and invites participants to discuss each of the questions. Often, the discussion can uncover the meanings and experiences common to all participants that would not be learned from individual interviews or surveys. This occurs when, during the discussion, participants are reminded of things they had not thought of initially. It is the group dynamics that often helps bring out new insights and provides a deeper analysis of the situation. Focus groups are often used in conjunction with surveys to "dig down" deeper into the survey results, which helps to explain these results in more detail. Krueger and Casey (2014) provide a good resource for focus group approaches.

Participant observation and nonparticipant observation can also be used to understand a particular event. In participant observation, the program evaluator is immersed and part of the team to seek a clearer understanding as a working member of the team. In a nonparticipant observational situation, the teamwork might be observed but is done externally, such as reviewing a videotaped session.

Mixed Methods Strategies

Mixed method strategies are just what the name implies—they are any combination of qualitative and quantitative approaches. For example, the evaluation team may use a survey and then conduct a focus group to better understand the survey results. In many instances, surveys give the broad picture of a situation. Conversely, the focus group through "focused" questions can pinpoint and specify the experience so that the evaluator has a greater understanding of the phenomenon. Another example would be to use a nonstructured observation instrument with a videotaped session followed by a live debriefing session. Similar to the preceding example, the debriefing session might provide a more in-depth interpretation of what was observed using the nonstructured observation. In both of the examples listed earlier, the purpose of the mixed method strategy is to be as pragmatic as possible to get a greater understanding of the dynamics of the interprofessional project being evaluated. Box 11.2 describes the implementation and evaluation of an IPE program.

BOX 11.2

Implementation and Evaluation of an Interprofessional Education Program: An Exemplar

Dr. A and Dr. R were medical and nursing faculty members at a major academic health center containing a hospital, a medical school, a nursing program, and health professional programs in occupational therapy, physical therapy, and pharmacy, among others. They had been friends for several years and had worked together on various projects in the past. Recently, they had attended a few professional meetings and listened to several presentations about interprofessional education (IPE) programs at other universities. Both of them were impressed with the success of these programs. They also began to believe that care delivery in the future would rely on teams. Because of this, they were convinced that their students would need to be prepared for this change. At one professional meeting, they discussed their interest over coffee and began to brainstorm about a program that might be appropriate at their university. They outlined some components of a potential program and discussed the idea with some of their colleagues when they returned to their university. They found that many of the faculty agreed that an IPE program would be beneficial to their students. They then discussed their interest with their respective deans and found that the deans also shared their belief about the needed changes. Both deans suggested that they determine the interest level of faculty in their departments and that of the faculty in the other health professions programs. The deans indicated that if there were sufficient interest and if they could put together a reasonable plan, they would take the proposal to the president.

Encouraged by the deans' responses, they scanned the literature and then surveyed faculty in the programs. The faculty survey results showed that several faculty members were interested in being involved in a program that would advance IPE. They then convened a working group with representatives from all of the programs to brainstorm what a program would look like. After reviewing the results from the literature search, the group started by defining the goals of the proposed program. They decided, since the concept of IPE was so new to students, that it would be important to have students develop a positive attitude toward the concept. To do this, they designed a project that was intended to introduce students to the concept of interprofessional care. They would then assess student attitudes at the beginning and end of the project. From the literature review, they had found an attitude survey called the *Interdisciplinary Education Perception Scale* (IEPS), which was a validated instrument being used by numerous programs. They reviewed the instrument and believed that it was the appropriate one to use and that a measure of effectiveness would be a significant increase in attitude score from the beginning to the end. They also believed that since an important audience for the results was the president and deans, showing positive student attitudes would help in getting their support to continue and develop a more comprehensive program.

With these decisions made, they agreed that any project needed to involve all students and should be required. They also believed that it should be lengthy enough so that real learning could occur. With input from all members of the group and support of the deans, they put together a year-long project consisting of various interprofessional activities requiring students to work in teams. Students were also given team assignments. The project was submitted and approved by the president, and the first cohort of students began. They surveyed the students at the beginning of the project and found what they considered some relatively positive attitudes about IPE. Many of the activities seemed to work very well during the year, and most of the assignments were completed on time and fairly well. In some of the meetings that they held with students, they heard some complaints about time commitments and that some students were not contributing enough to the team assignments. At the end of the year, they surveyed students with the IEPS again. Although the results showed some significant differences between professions, there were no significant increases from the pretest. In fact, the mean attitudes

BOX 11.2

Implementation and Evaluation of an Interprofessional Education Program: An Exemplar (*continued*)

of some professions actually decreased slightly. This obviously caused some concern among the team, and they decided to dig deeper to find out why some of the attitudes declined. They reviewed the team assignments and talked to student leaders. They also asked students to participate in a series of focus groups to discuss the strengths and weaknesses of the project. The students told them that they enjoyed meeting students in the other professions and had learned a lot about what they did. However, they thought that the team assignments were just "busy work" and did not really relate to the activities. They also thought that some members of their team were not serious about the assignments and did not contribute very much. Thus, it was not the substantive part of the project that was causing problems but more of the administrative requirements. With this formative evaluation information in mind, the team made some modifications to the assignments so that they had a more direct relationship to each of the activities. They then set up a peer evaluation system so that each member of the team could evaluate other members. They also set up an advisory committee of student leaders to work closely with the faculty team. In this way, they would be able to learn if there were other problems occurring that might lessen the effect of the team training. These changes seemed to have a positive effect on student attitudes, as they began to see some noticeable improvements over the next two cohorts of students participating in the project. With these positive results in hand, they submitted the description of the project and the evaluation results for presentation at their professional conferences and continued to gather feedback. As a result of the ongoing feedback, they began working on a more comprehensive IPE program for all students.

DISSEMINATION

As noted previously, simply conducting and evaluating an IPE project is not enough. Sharing the lessons learned in the development, implementation, and evaluation of IPE initiatives is also important. Presenting at conferences via podium or poster sessions and publishing in peer-reviewed journals or newsletters are some examples of ways to disseminate the results of IPE projects or IPE curriculum evaluation. Additionally, creating a dissemination plan that includes both experts and novice members encourages teamwork as they collaborate on how to showcase their projects.

Newsletters

The first and relatively easiest approach to dissemination would be to write a short piece on the results of the evaluation of your project for a newsletter. Most universities have in-house newsletters, as do local or national professional associations. Most newsletter editors and editorial boards are looking for short articles that might be of interest to the readership. The articles should contain a simple description of the nature of the project, how it was evaluated, and the results of the evaluation. These short pieces can also serve as a head start on writing a longer article for a professional journal and can serve as an abstract to submit for presentation at a local or national conference.

Conferences

Local, national and international conferences provide a greater way to communicate with a larger audience. For the novice, local conferences are a good way to gain experience, as they have acceptance criteria that are often a little less rigorous than those of national conferences. Usually about 6 to 8 months prior to the conference, the association will publish a call for abstracts that contains directions for submitting an application along with a detailed list of specific information that will need to be included. Many will also contain the abstract submission criteria that are used by the conference evaluators and list criteria that describes the variety of presentation formats. Subsequently, conference dissemination can be a valuable opportunity to gain experience and professional growth, get feedback on the IPE project presented, network with other professionals who have similar interests, and help foster career growth and opportunities for collaborative projects.

Journal Articles

Journal articles are the way to reach the largest number of people, especially when written for national or international journals. Getting an article published in a journal gives the IPE project and subsequent evaluation "staying power," since once it is in print, it can be accessed by others for years. Whereas a presentation at a conference may have an impact just at the conference, a published article has the potential for long-term impact. Drafting conference presentations can provide the framework and outline for a journal article. As with conferences, there are journals with a more local flavor, whereas others are more national or international in scope. Before deciding on a journal, it is important to match journal emphasis with writing experience and the manuscript focus. Tips for getting published are presented in Figure 11.3 and described more fully in the following.

First, read the journal so that you can understand the types of articles it publishes, and note whether they tend to be heavily research oriented or more descriptive. Consider

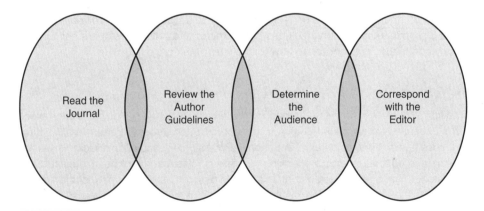

FIGURE 11.3 Tips for Getting Published.

the style of writing of the articles: Are they more or less formal? Is the targeted audience faculty, researchers, or clinicians?

Second, locate the author guidelines, and follow them closely. Adhering to the rules of the journal will help in getting published, as the editor may just reject it during the editor's review and not send it out to the peer reviewers.

Third, understand whether the readership is faculty, researchers, or clinicians, as these are the people deciding whether the manuscript will be published. It is important that the manuscript is clear and concise: Good writing will not overcome a poor idea, but poor writing can sabotage a good one. Reviewers are busy people and are reviewing manuscripts as a professional courtesy. Thus, it is important not to force them to search for main ideas or to be distracted by typographical errors or poorly constructed sentences.

Finally, work with the editor. He or she can be helpful regarding whether the manuscript is appropriate for the journal and in many cases will review a brief abstract of the manuscript, note if it is an appropriate fit, and even make some suggestions about what it would need to be acceptable. It is important to note that similarly to author guidelines, editor suggestions should be followed.

Additionally, be aware of four other considerations in submitting an article for publication. The first is that once a manuscript is submitted, it may take up to a year for it to appear in print. This is because of the time given to reviewers to critique it and for authors to make necessary revisions. Once accepted, it may be another 3 to 6 months before the article is published, as most journals have numerous articles waiting for publication. Note that a publishing fee can be common. Finally, manuscripts cannot be submitted simultaneously to multiple journals, as once your manuscript is accepted, the journal owns the copyright of the article.

IMPLICATIONS FOR NURSING PRACTICE

Evaluating IPE projects and disseminating the results has some important implications for nursing practice. As noted throughout the book, the future of nursing is inextricably tied to interprofessional care, and students need to be prepared to function as part of an interprofessional team. Providing successful interprofessional experiences is critical in nursing education, and evaluation of these experiences is the only way to know what is successful. Nursing students should have exposure to and experience with interprofessional teams. They need to understand the components of effective teamwork and then gain practical experience working as part of a team. This suggests that both didactic and clinical experiences, as outlined in Chapters 6 through 8, should be an integral part of the nursing program. Although many students come to their educational program with some understanding of teamwork through athletic or other types of experiences, working in a healthcare setting with individuals from different disciplines requires them to gain additional skills and learn to be a productive member of a healthcare team. Three types of nursing student experiences, explained in the following sections, might help to prepare them for success in the evolving healthcare system in which they will practice: didactic, observational, and hands-on. It is also important to reiterate that evaluating each of these experiences is crucial to maximizing their effectiveness.

Didactic Experiences

Didactic experiences might include classroom experiences, preferably with students from other disciplines, to discuss and understand the importance of interprofessional approaches to care. These learning activities might include those in which students work together on projects to help them understand the roles and responsibilities of those in other disciplines. Most students in the health professions come to their educational programs with stereotypical views of other professions, if they have any understanding at all.

Helping nursing students understand what skills other professionals have will help them understand and respect the contributions that these professionals can make to patient care. Other classroom activities involving students working on simulated activities can add to their appreciation of the necessity of working in teams and the potential contributions of other professions. One major focus on the evaluation of these didactic experiences should then be on the extent to which students come to understand and value the contribution of other professions in the delivery of care. Another focus during this period might be on improving their attitudes toward working in teams. Survey instruments such as the IEPS, possibly along with focus groups, should provide an assessment of the effectiveness of these activities in enhancing student attitudes toward other professions and teamwork.

Observational Experiences

Observing effective teams in action can give students an understanding of the behaviors that constitute effective team functioning. These observations can be through videotaped sessions or observing real teams in action. Using a simple observation instrument, such as the JTOG (described earlier), that directs students' attention to effective behaviors can enable students to see concrete examples of these behaviors. After the observation, an important activity is to debrief as a team about what was observed. In addition to debriefing sessions, having students reflect on and write down what they learned from the various scenarios is another important approach to helping them understand how effective teams operate. These experiences can pave the way for students to begin working in actual teams and knowing the kinds of behaviors that lead to effective teamwork.

Hands-On Experiences

The most critical component of preparing students to work in teams is to actually work in a clinical setting as a member of a team. This can be accomplished by having students work as a team, under the guidance of clinical mentors, with real patients. One approach that can be successful is to have each student review a particular patient's chart from his or her discipline-specific perspective and come together under an experienced mentor to discuss the case, possibly visit with the patient as a team, and then come together again and debrief the situation and come up with a plan of care. Having students conduct self-evaluation of their behavior during these activities or engaging in peer assessments can be powerful ways to improve performance. Often, because of scheduling problems, it is difficult to find times in which students can come together. With the advent of more sophisticated technology (as described in Chapter 9), it is now possible to bring individuals together via computer applications during these sessions. Case study analysis is another example of hands-on experience. Students can work together over a period of time on various interprofessional activities or with standardized or simulated patients. Evaluating these experiences through debriefing activities, reflection papers, focus groups, or self- and peer evaluation activities are all valuable ways to learn the effectiveness of these activities in teaching the concepts of interprofessional collaboration.

CONCLUSION

The essence of evaluating IPE programs and then the value of disseminating the results is important when creating an IPE and/or CP project. As noted, providing nursing students with an opportunity to engage in interprofessional learning experiences prepares them to work as an effective member of the team. Just as engaging students in these team experiences is vital to building a workforce able to provide patient-centered care, so is the value and need to evaluate these initiatives for their effectiveness. This can only be accomplished by having a framework containing well-tested concepts by which to guide student learning and the delivery of care. Development of this framework can be accomplished at the local level by rigorous evaluation of projects and programs aimed at identifying the common core principles of IPE. This chapter described the major components of a program evaluation in a step-by-step manner, identifying the why, what, and how of evaluation, and classified the key components of an evaluation plan, emphasizing the importance of identifying clear, measurable goals built into an IPE program during the planning stage. The "what" and the "how" of IPE evaluation, as well as measurement methods, were described, and an exemplar of how these might be carried out in an educational setting was provided.

Since sharing successful program and project outcomes at professional conferences or in professional journals is vital to the advancement of IPE, this chapter discussed and explored various dissemination methods and modalities. IPE and CP must be a critical component of nursing education if nurse educators are going to prepare their students for a healthcare system that uses team-based patient-centered care approaches. To that end, this chapter included some examples of experiences to help nursing students develop skills in interprofessional teamwork and how the effectiveness of these experiences might be evaluated.

References

Barnstable, S. (2003). *Nurse as educator: Principles of teaching and learning for nursing practice* (2nd ed.). Sudbury, MA: Jones & Bartlett.

Canadian Interprofessional Health Collaborative. (2012). *An inventory of quantitative tools to measure interprofessional education and collaborative practice.* Vancouver, BC: Author. Available at http://rcrc.brandeis.edu

Freeth, D. (2001). Sustaining interprofessional collaboration. *Journal of Interprofessional Care, 15*(1), 37–46.

Freeth, D., Hammick, M., Koppel, I., Reeves, S., & Barr, H. (2002). *A critical review of evaluations of interprofessional education.* London: LTSN Health Sciences and Practice.

Heinemann, G. D., Schmitt, M. H., Farrell, M. P., & Brallier, S. A., (1999). Development of an Attitudes Toward Health Care Teams Scale. *Evaluation and the Health Professions, 22,* 123–142.

Humphris, D., & Hean, S. (2004). Educating the future workforce: Building the evidence about interprofessional learning. *Journal of Health Services Research and Policy, 9*(Suppl. 1), 24–27.

Institute of Medicine. (2013). *Measuring the impact of interprofessional education on collaborative practice and patient outcomes.* Washington, DC: National Academies Press.

Interprofessional Education Collaborative Expert Panel. (2011). *Core competencies for interprofessional collaborative practice: Report of an expert panel.* Washington, DC: Interprofessional Education Collaborative.

Jefferson Center for Interprofessional Education. (2016). *Jefferson Teamwork Observation Guide.* Available at http://www.jefferson.edu/university/interprofessional_education.html

Johnson, T. P. (2014). *Handbook of health survey methods.* Wiley Handbooks in Survey Methodology. Available at http://www.researchandmarkets.com/publication/mz1riqk/handbook_of_health_survey

Krueger R. A., & Casey M. A. (2014). *Focus groups: A practical guide for applied research* (5th ed.). Thousand Oaks, CA: Sage.

Luecht, R. M., Madsen, M. K., Taugher, M. P., & Petterson, B. J. (1990). Assessing professional perceptions: Design and validation of an Interdisciplinary Education Perception Scale. *Journal of Allied Health, 19*(1), 181–191.

National Center for Interprofessional Practice and Education. (2015). Home page. Retrieved June 8, 2016, from https://www.nexusipe.org

Pollard, K. C., & Miers, M. E. (2008). From students to professionals: Results of a longitudinal study of attitudes to pre-qualifying collaborative learning and working in health and social care in the United Kingdom. *Journal of Interprofessional Care, 22*(4), 399–416.

Reeves, S., Perrier, L., Goldman, J., Freeth, D., & Zwarenstein, M. (2013). *Training health and social care professionals to work together.* London: Cochrane Collaboration.

Schofield, R., & Amodeo, M. (1999). Interdisciplinary teams in health care and human services: Are they effective? *Health and Social Work, 24,* 210–219.

Stone, N. (2006). Evaluating interprofessional education: The tautological need for interdisciplinary approaches. *Journal of Interprofessional Care, 20*(3), 260–275.

Tashakkori, A., & Creswell, J. (2007). The new era of mixed methods. *Journal of Mixed Methods Research, 1*(1), 3–8.

World Health Organization. (2010). *Framework for action on interprofessional education and collaborative practice.* Geneva, Switzerland: Author. Available at http://apps.who.int/iris/bitstream/10665/70185/1/WHO_HRH_HPN_10.3_eng.pdf

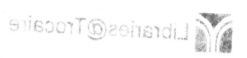

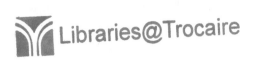